We're Surviving Cancer . . . Today

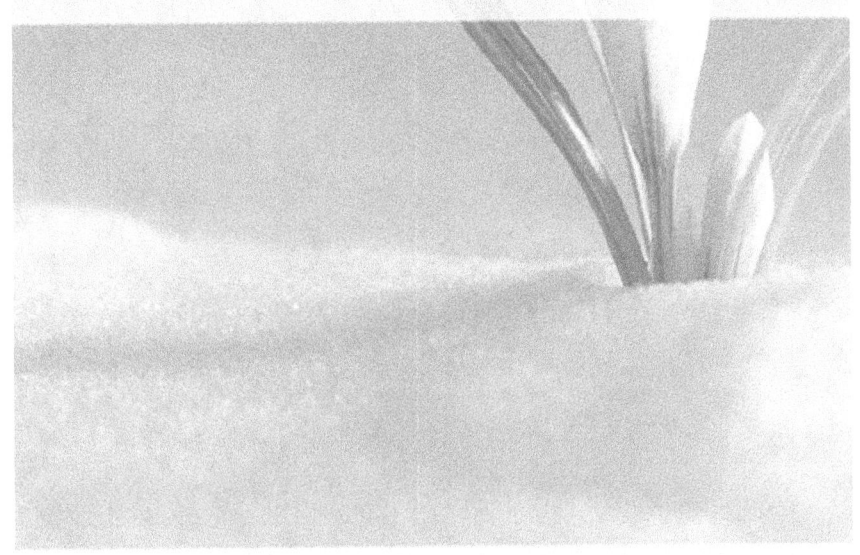

Bennett Lentczner
and
Linda Whitesitt

DEDICATION

To all our family and friends who continue to help us survive.

CONTENTS

ACKNOWLEDGMENTS

We thank all of the doctors and health care practitioners who have applied their expertise and experience in providing diagnoses, advice and appropriate treatments. Most importantly, we are grateful to all of them for speaking truth so that we can continue to make decisions that balance quality of living with quantity of life.

Dr. Paul Quarantillo, III, Family Practitioner, Berkeley Springs, WV
Dr. Shane Geib, Urologist, Winchester, VA
Dr. Edward Kiggundu, Radiation Oncologist, Martinsburg, WV
Dr. Jeffrey Lessar, Pulmonologist, Winchester, VA
Dr. David Drake, Plastic Surgeon, University of Virginia, Charlottesville, VA
Dr. Bruce Flax, Radiation Oncologist, Winchester, VA
Dr. Ejaz Kahn, Electrophysiologist, Winchester, VA
Dr. Issac Mathai, Holistic Medicine, Bangalore, India
Michael Pushkin, Massage Therapist, Berkeley Springs, WV
Tamme Marggraf, Acupuncturist, Berkeley Springs, WV
Peter Juergensen, Clinical Orthopedic Massage Therapist, Martinsburg, WV
Dr. Brian S. Erickson, D.C., Shepherdstown, WV
Rev. Edward L. "Red" Duke, Ft. Lauderdale, FL
Lydia Walker, LPC, Berkeley Springs, WV
Dana Dales, PMP, Berkeley Springs, WV
Sandra Kay, LPC, Berkeley Springs, WV
Lisa Rader, A-NP, Winchester, VA

Special gratitude to . . .

Dr. Benjamin Kozower, Thoracic and Cardiovascular Surgeon, University of Virginia, Charlottesville, VA
and
Dr. William Houck, III, Oncologist, Winchester, VA

We extend our appreciation to all of the nurses and office personnel who support these fine caregivers and offer us the benefit of their heartfelt comfort and concern.

INTRODUCTION

We know we're showing our age, but both of us are startled when someone comments "We're having a baby!" Our silent reaction is "How can 'we' – two people – have a baby?" We appreciate the reason behind the "we," but we still can't help being surprised by the first person plural pronoun and awed that in using "we," the speaker has chosen to honor the role that both parents have in the baby-making and baby-having process.

Thinking about the "we're having a baby" announcement, we've come to realize that we would like to borrow the first person plural pronoun when talking about how we live with Bennett's cancer. If Linda says "my husband is surviving cancer," she feels missing from that announcement, just like in the past when one of the partners in the baby-making process was left out when the other partner said, "I'm having a baby!" It is important to both of us that Linda is included in Bennett's journey of surviving cancer. Every day, every moment, it takes two of us to survive.

We're also using the phrase "we're surviving cancer" rather than "we are a cancer survivor." Not only is there a lack of agreement between "we" and "a cancer survivor," but in our experience with

Bennett's multiple battles with cancer – prostate, lung cancer and the recurrence of lung cancer – there has never been a time when it has felt like the "cancer chapter" has been completely closed. It has always been much more of a feeling of "today we're surviving cancer, tomorrow who knows."

In the fall of 2011 we learned that Bennett's lung cancer had recurred. Could we still talk about "we're surviving cancer"? We felt that we could. In fact, we felt that we must. It's what kept us going. For today, we are surviving; by tonight, we will have survived the day; by tomorrow, we pray that we will have survived as well.

In this book we do not write about how to survive cancer and live happily ever after. We don't know how to do that. Rather, we tell our stories about how "we're surviving cancer . . . today." In Bennett's story of his day-to-day survival, he draws from the periodic health updates he has sent to family and friends. These messages have allowed those who care about him to become intimate members of a loving, extended support network that has provided Bennett with enormous amounts of spiritual and healing energy. He hopes his story will help others understand the benefit of not carrying the burden of anxiety alone and the advantage of sharing joy and despair with those who offer love and support.

Linda's story is a collection of reflections on how she has navigated the terrain of surviving cancer with Bennett and where she has found the inspiration and strength to continue their journey. She hopes her words will help others walk the path with a loved one who is surviving cancer one day at a time.

Both of us hope that the love we have for each other as well as the love our friends and family have offered us throughout this journey shines through every page. It is that love that has carried us across the hills and valleys of our surviving cancer journey, giving us the hope and courage to face every day.

BENNETT'S STORY

I write not to suggest that I am some kind of brave hero in a fight for survival with cancer, but rather to share my experiences, insights and feelings and to offer some thoughts that hopefully might help others traveling this road. I know that there are many whose journeys have been much more difficult than mine. Hearing their stories and reading the words of others who have had to face adversity have helped me more than all of the books I've collected with recipes for diets and lifestyle changes that promote ways of surviving with cancer. I don't want to suggest that such books and CDs are not helpful – they are and have been for me, providing much useful information about nurturing my body. But more important are the stories of those who have been on this journey. They have helped me learn that human beings are capable of accepting profound challenges and, for some period of time, sustaining a full life.

The experience of cancer has brought me face to face with the hardest reality we all must face: no one gets out of this life alive. I don't want to imply that facing this reality is in any way easy, but once we accept this simple fact, no matter what one's religious beliefs are in this regard, we can go forward for whatever time we have here, ensuring time for love and humor. As a very wise older gentleman told me at the start of a round of golf on a rather cloudy, drizzly day, "This is a great day! I am on this side of the grass!"

I began my relationship with cancer through the experiences I had with family and friends who were dealing with cancer. I lost both my mother and sister to lung cancer. In retrospect I know that I learned much from them as I watched each of them confront cancer. My mother never lost her love of life. For her, the journey was all about the quality of life as she continued to play golf and enjoy her friends and family, especially her children and grandchildren. She accepted the path she had been placed on with grace, optimism and humor.

My sister did not have an easy journey with cancer. It began shortly after she had retired and moved from New York to Florida where she was just starting to enjoy a good life in a warm climate. For most of her journey she was angry and frustrated with what the cancer and the treatments were doing to her. While her feelings were understandable, it was extremely hard for all of us to watch her struggle in her final days.

At the beginning of my own cancer journey – when I was told that I had prostate cancer – I had not yet processed the contrasting lessons of my mother's and sister's journeys. Nor had I thought about how others I knew who had faced cancer had dealt with it. I'm afraid my initial reactions to hearing I had cancer were probably typical of many upon hearing the "C" word applied to themselves – fear and anger, dread and sadness, anxiety and self-pity – why me? Little did I know then just how extensive and varied my journey with cancer was going to be and, even more importantly, how strong I would become through the love and support of my wife, children, family and friends. I would be less than truthful if I wrote that I have never doubted the outcome of my journey, never felt that I could not find the energy to continue the battles, and never felt that it was time to meet the inevitable departure from this life on earth. I cannot say for certain what it is within me that continues to propel me along the path of living to the fullest every day, but I do know that I have chosen the path my mother took – optimism, humor, believing in something bigger than myself, and an emphasis on the quality of my life not the quantity of years I might simply be alive.

My life has been shaped by a drive to succeed in order to please my father. It took the help of a very skilled counselor to help me realize that what I felt as his demand for excellence was his way of expressing his love for me – making me reach to be all I could be all of the time. It is a trait that I inherited, making demands on my students to become all they could become. This drive to succeed has caused me to push on because I have not yet reached the point when I can say to my father, "This is all I can be – this is all I can do." At the age of 75, I have no idea when I will know that point, only that I trust he will let me know, and I will be OK with that. In the meantime, I appreciate having the energy that comes from meeting his expectations to help me not only fight my cancers, but learn to accept each new episode as yet another challenge in fulfilling my life.

Over the past four years I have experienced prostate cancer, lung cancer, and a recurrence of lung cancer. In 2008, I had brachytherapy followed by direct beam radiation treatments for the prostate cancer. In the summer of 2009, I was diagnosed with lung cancer. That September, the lower third of my right lung was removed, and the surgery was followed by chemotherapy to promote non-recurrence of the cancer. Two years later a CT scan revealed three metastatic lymph nodes behind my esophagus. Treatment was begun in late December 2011 – seven weeks of radiation and chemotherapy. By March a CT scan showed no evidence of cancer anywhere, and as of this writing, I remain cancer free.

I keep living my life doing all of things that matter to me. I am a trumpet player, and while the loss of a portion of my right lung and the more recently discovered scarring in the same lung has greatly reduced my capacity for air, I keep playing and by all reports from my colleagues, playing acceptably. I continue to enjoy one or two rounds of golf every week, and I work at our local golf course as a starter.

It is always a relief to get what my oncologist calls "boring CT scan reports" – reports that indicate nothing other than a good, healthy, cancer- free body. The truth is I find it difficult to live from CT scan to CT scan. My wife and I enjoy eleven weeks of not thinking about the next scan followed by a week of wondering what the scan might reveal and then several anxious days waiting to visit the oncologist to receive the report. This schedule notwithstanding, we remain positive about my life and grateful for the time we share in good health and spirit. The calendar is just a reminder that once you experience cancer, your life changes. I am among the lucky ones – my life continues with wonderful quality.

I truly believe that the communication with friends and family that I have carried on along with my wife, Linda, and my daughter, Julie, during the course of my journey with cancer was, and continues to be, of immeasurable importance in helping us through each part of this journey. Using CarePages, a service of the University of Virginia Medical Center, I have been able to post and share comments about my journey and, more importantly, gather much healing and spiritual energy. It has become the primary home of my cancer support group. Much of what I have learned about myself has come through these writings. Because of the interactivity of the communication, we have been surrounded by those who care as well as some who are willing to share their own experiences and feelings. There have been 102 participants in this support group alone.

Like many who read this book, we have many friends who are shy of subscribing to anything on the Internet. At the request of these dear and caring friends and relatives, I post my CarePages messages on my Facebook page and send them in group emails. This comprehensive sharing brings the number of family, friends and former students to close to 200. I have been humbled by their continuing concern and good wishes as well as buoyed by the healing energy they send to me with each new posting.

If you are like me, it is relatively easy to share a narrative about your physical condition; it is not so easy to share your feelings, anxieties or fears about that condition. My hope is that the readers of my story will gain insight into how to share their journey with those who care about them. My experience has shown me that there are untold numbers of people who appreciate the opportunity to listen and provide support. Don't assume they don't want to be bothered. Do presume that they care and give them a chance to say so. Suffice it to say that the process of writing news and feelings – good and not so good – reveals one's inner-most feelings and attitudes. Writing, when allowed to originate from deep within, can strip out the buried "bad" so that it does not detract from the challenges of today's survival. The process of openly sharing helps replace fear with hope, and anxiety with optimism and humor. These are powerful healers.

My postings did not begin until I was well down the path on our cancer journey – almost four weeks after the initial lung surgery. At those times when I felt alone, I had only to read the messages sent to me by family and friends. Their words got me through many a difficult hour. (I have not included the responses to each of the postings because of their personal nature.)

The original surgery to remove what was believed to be a small spot of cancer from my right lung was to be performed thoracoscopically. The surgeon Dr. Benjamin Kozower (University of Virginia) had to delay the procedure at the last minute because his first child – a son – decided to enter the world on the day I was to have my operation. The surgery was delayed and took place ten days later. I went under anesthesia with the thought that this was going to be a relatively simple procedure. It was not. Early in the operation Dr. Kozower discovered a lymph node "he did not like the looks of," and when the biopsy showed it to be malignant, he opened me up and removed an additional twenty-five lymph nodes he suspected could be involved. (Fortunately, none of them showed any evidence of cancer.) When I was able to understand the severity of the surgery, I asked Dr. Kozower two questions: would I be able to play the trumpet again and would I be around for his newborn son's Bar Mitzvah. He answered "yes" to both questions. I said my only remaining question was would I be invited to the Bar Mitzvah. His response – "absolutely!" I then promised to play at his son's Bar Mitzvah. This is a promise I intend to keep!

About four weeks after the initial surgery, I "sprung a leak," as Dr. Kozower would later explain. This is a rare and serious complication from lung surgery. After a night of ambulance rides and emergency rooms, I was transported back to UVA and

Dr. Kozower's care. It was during that stay at UVA Medical Center that we became aware of CarePages.

What follows is an edited selection of postings from October 4, 2009 to the present. Beginning in 2011 these messages were also shared in emails and on Facebook. Some of the postings were written by my wife and daughter. Together with my introductions to the entries (printed in italics), they provide a journal of my roller coaster journey and insights into how I find day-to-day survival possible.

I frequently review my journey – our journey – to make sure that I am listening to my body, keeping my mind on a positive path, honoring the universe, and accepting the energy sent as love, prayers and healing by the many who circle to protect me. Remembering how this journey began renews my faith in living today.

Second Lung Surgery

*My condition after the surgery to fix the leak in my lung was extremely weak.
These postings by Linda and Julie describe what transpired and how I responded
to treatment, all of which was traumatic for everyone, including Dr. Kozower. In
Linda's story found later in this book, she also describes the night before this
surgery and how my roommate managed to move his bed closer to mine, hold my
hand while I wept in pure fear, and pray for and with me.*

October 4, 2009 5:56 pm

Dr. Kozower said that Bennett's surgery went well. It started around
10 am and took 3 ½ hours. He located the tiny hole at the bottom of
the middle lobe, applied a patch using a cow membrane (we're going
to call his lung "Bessie"), and then had a plastic surgeon (Dr. Drake)
move the serratus muscle over the patch. According to Dr. Kozower,
all of it looked good.

He had to reopen Bennett's long incision and insert three
drainage tubes. Bennett also has an IV line in his neck. Tomorrow
they will install a picc line in his upper left arm so the nurses don't
have to keep sticking him for blood or IV.

As I'm writing this, Bennett said to tell you – "I shot an 87 today
. . . and then I played the second hole." He still has his sense of
humor, helped undoubtedly by the morphine and other pain
medications.

The doctors and nurses are being terrific as usual. Bennett's
roommate/buddy went home today, but he waited around to find out
about Bennett's surgery. He's a dear, sweet man, and he plans on
coming to visit Bennett this week.

Dr. Kozower anticipates that Bennett will be in the hospital for a week or more and will not send him home until we are all comfortable with Bennett being three hours away from UVA. – Linda

October 5, 2009 5:01 pm

Bennett has been moved to a private room, and he walked to get there. He is still on a liquid diet until his nausea subsides. He has regained his sense of humor as evidenced by his stories for the medical staff that come in and, more importantly, he has found the strength to start fighting. The resounding message that I (Julie) hear is, "If anyone can beat this, it's Bennett." Very true!

Dr. Kozower has visited Dad twice today and told him that he is happy to see him doing so well. I was truly touched when he told Dad that on Saturday he actually lost sleep worrying about him. But tonight Dr. Kozower will sleep peacefully and so will we. We really feel like Dr. Kozower is more than just a brilliant surgeon – he is a part of our circle of friends and family.

Linda is doing much better now that Dad is on the right path again. She and I enjoyed a nice Thai dinner and a bottle of wine. She got a good night's sleep and woke up this morning with a newfound appreciation for a good night's sleep.

Thank you everyone for being a part of our circle – a circle that has no beginning and no end of love for my family. – Julie

From Linda – it is so good to see Bennett up and around with great color in his cheeks! When the nurse had him sniff an alcohol patch this morning because he felt faint, he told her that he'd take an olive with it! Bennett dictating to Julie – To all of my supporters: It sure was crowded in my operating room yesterday with all of you there. I so appreciate ALL of you and the love and prayers that you bring to me in this difficult time in my life. As I sit – yes, sit in my hospital room – I know that it would not be possible for me to have the strength this new surgery requires without each and every one of you at my side. So please know that all of this is simply a slight detour to the mid-80's . . . FORE!!!

October 6, 2009 5:40 pm

Bennett is a real trooper! After a difficult night last night (he got behind in controlling the pain), he's made steady improvement all day. But lest all of you think he's ready to play golf, he says that it'll be at least a week or two before he can even look at a golf club.

His wonderful nurse has had him walking several times today and sitting up in the chair most of the day. She is fantastic with him – gentle, loving and encouraging! Dr. Kozower is pleased with his progress, particularly how much better Bennett looked this afternoon.

Thank you for your messages and emails. They continue to lift our spirits! – Linda

October 7, 2009 6:33 pm

Bennett struggled with nausea and a reaction to medication today (tremors and difficulty breathing). Benadryl seemed to help the reaction, and his nurse is trying a different anti-nausea medication. Dr. Kozower ordered a brain and chest CT scan just to check, although he doesn't expect to find anything.

We brought in some miso soup that so far has set well on Bennett's tummy, and he ate a little Jell-O. Right now he's awake enough to watch the Yankees.

We're learning to breathe deeply when going over these unexpected bumps in the road. As the charge nurse says, Bennett has been through quite a lot, and it will take time and persistence to heal. – Linda

October 8, 2009 7:16 pm

Every hour brings something new. Sometimes we're taking steps forward and sometimes not.

Bennett's nausea is somewhat better as is his pain. He has a spasm in a vein in his arm that caused it to swell and be painful. They checked for blood clots – nothing.

We just finished dinner – miso soup from a local restaurant, and we are about take a stroll down the hall.

Many thanks to all of you for your wonderful good wishes, jokes, prayers, affirmations, and words of encouragement.

Julie went home to family today – our grandson needs his mommy. We miss her, but we know that she's with us and walking the same path as we are.

Big important news from Bennett tonight – in his words, "I pooped." He hopes that the systems are "all go" from now on. – Linda

October 9, 2009 7:00 pm

The roller coaster continues to go up and down on an hourly basis, but overall, I think it's calming down. The doctor is trying to get Bennett off all of the meds except for the pain medication in an attempt to reduce his hallucinations. Bennett spent much time last night talking to people who were not in the room and eating and drinking stuff that didn't exist. He would awaken quite confused. The doctor is convinced that the medication is the cause. Chemicals –

how amazing they are. He needs them for pain and to prevent infection, but unfortunately they cause strange reactions.

He had two more tubes taken out today, leaving two more to go. He is so much more comfortable.

Right now, he's watching the Yankees (thanks to all of you Yankee supporters out there).

We couldn't make it through all of this without every one of you. It's hard to believe that he's been here a week. But to put that in perspective, his new roommate has been here for six weeks! I can't even begin to imagine. – Linda

October 10, 2009 6:56 pm

We're tired. Bennett's tired. We want to go home. Complaining is good for the soul. Thanks for listening. – Linda

October 11, 2009 1:16 pm

Today is not only a gorgeous day filled with beautiful fall colors and a golden sun, but a day truly to be grateful. Linda just called me and she was on I-81 bringing Daddy home.

All the tubes are OUT! The only medication he is on is for pain (Vicadin), and all signs point to healing. It has been said that the best healing is done at home. How exciting to believe that his healing will be twice as powerful now that they are back in Berkeley Springs.

On Thursday Linda will take Dad back to UVA to meet with Dr. Drake, the plastic surgeon. This is a follow-up visit to make sure that his work is healing the way it should. As Linda said, she doesn't mind making that trip since she knows she can take him home the same day.

This message board has been a wonderful tool to keep you posted and also to receive your many prayers, thoughts and loving wishes of good health. We will continue to utilize this to provide updates and receive your messages. However, now that he is home and Linda is focused on him more than ever, these updates won't be every day.

You have ALL been a light to our family and bring joy with every message you send. Through each step, whether big or small, they walk this healing journey with grace, FAITH, love and strength. We celebrate today and every day and know in our hearts that Bennett is a fighter, and as many of you have said, "if anyone can beat this, it is Bennett."

Thank you all and may your days be filled with many blessings. – Julie

October 14, 2009 1:57 pm

We thank all of you for your wonderful welcome home messages. It is so great to be home! Bennett is getting a little stronger all the time. We are definitely going in the right direction this time. – Linda

October 18, 2009 5:26 pm

Bennett continues to get a little stronger every day. We are so grateful that everything seems to be going well.

Jeffrey, Bennett's "adopted" son from NY, surprised us by showing up on our doorstep at 8:00 am last Thursday to take us to Charlottesville for Bennett's doctor's appointment. What a guy! It was wonderful to have him here -- it gave me the chance to get out and do some errands. Thanks, Jeff!

The plastic surgeon thought Bennett was doing very well, and he was impressed with Bennett's range of motion. He indicated that it would be two to four months before he considered Bennett "out of the woods," but he seemed to be pleased with the progress so far. It will take that amount of time before he is certain that the patch will hold permanently.

Dr. Kozower called on Thursday to check on Bennett, and we have a nurse coming in several times to help with the wounds (stitches and staples come out tomorrow), check vitals and help us know that everything is progressing nicely.

Bennett walks through the house several times a day, is up to eat (his appetite is returning) and takes naps throughout the day. He would have preferred to sleep through the Giant's defeat today, but he's thrilled with the Yankees! – Linda

Next Phase: Chemotherapy

One month after the trauma of the second surgery I was home facing the next step in this journey. The experience of surviving what I truly believed would be the end of my life had somehow given me the confidence to go through whatever was advisable to assure living for as long as possible. Little did I know how difficult this would become. During the arduous next few months, I learned that having specific short-term measurable goals was extremely important to surviving on a day-to-day basis. I was determined to succeed, and I added the following quotation as a header on my CarePages. It is an affirmation by Michael Hayes Samuelson that was sent to me by my friend Antonia with whom I spoke about her own experience surviving cancer. (Note: Antonia had survived cancer for more than ten years. She died in a home accident in 2011.)

Message to any remaining cancer cells:

"You may not tread on my spirit,
You may not occupy my soul."

November 1, 2009 7:49 am

This update is from ME. Yeah! I saw Dr. Kozower in Charlottesville on Thursday. After looking at my chest X-ray he said that everything looked good. He has now arranged for me to see an oncologist in Winchester. At that visit we will start to plan the chemo and radiation treatments.

Most importantly, Dr. K. gave me the go ahead to return to the trumpet. I have started doing about 10-15 minutes a day of long tones and easy modified scale exercises, playing softly. I can tell that my lung capacity is less, but that will improve as the healing continues.

I am walking more – about 0.35 miles per day. That is helping my legs feel stronger. Hope the weather cooperates so I can get outside every day. In the meantime, today I will be glued to the TV and the Giants. And tonight I am hopeful that the Yankees will make it 3-1!

November 15, 2009 12:49 pm

Hi everyone. I do want you to know how much your messages mean to me. They let me know that you are out there and care.

After much research and talking to people (including Dr. K who called from Charlottesville last Sunday evening), I, together with Linda, have decided to go ahead with the chemotherapy. We attended a class given by the oncology nurses, and it was helpful to meet them as well as others about to embark on this journey. I am following the advice of people I have spoken with and am determined that I will not get sick from these treatments.

Please keep me in your prayers and thoughts.

November 20, 2009 10:35 am

Yesterday we met with Dr. Houck, the oncologist. The chemotherapy sessions will be about 4 hours; the first session might be slightly longer because the nurses go over lots of info, etc. There will be 4 cycles of 21 days with treatment on day one of each cycle. For those who know something about chemo, I will be getting a combination of carboplatin, a fairly strong drug, and taxol.

My attitude remains quite positive. I have been bolstered by all of you, Dr. Houck and the nurses I have met in the oncology office. My return to all of the activities, family and friends that are so much a part of my life is imminent! Thanks for all of your messages and love. FORE!!!

November 21, 2009 3:50 pm

Just wanted you all to know how determined I am not to get sick from the chemo treatments. After talking with the head of the trumpet section of the Hagerstown Municipal Band (where I play all summer), I am planning to play rehearsals and in two holiday concerts in December.

How's that for a good note. :-) (As long as it is on the staff or below, I will be fine.)

November 25, 2009 12:34 pm

Yesterday went fine. I had no problems during the 5 ½ hour session and slept just fine last night. So far, today has been fine as well. I must share a motto I received from my avid supporter who went through this same chemo process 10 years ago. Many of you are old enough to remember where this comes from: "Better living through chemistry." It obviously worked for her, and it will work for me. Happy Thanksgiving to all of you.

November 30, 2009 8:07 am

You haven't heard from Bennett since last Wednesday because he's been dealing with the side effects of the first chemotherapy treatment. He was doing well until early afternoon on Thanksgiving, and then as he says, "the wheels came off the bus" – nausea, extreme fatigue, feeling like he had been hit by a very big bus. The nausea medication helps, but it makes him very sleepy. He just wants to go to sleep and wake up when this is all over – me, too! Hopefully, the worse will be over soon. They say that days 3-6 are usually pretty bad. He has received some homeopathic remedies from Dr. Mathai in India. Hopefully, they will help.

We hope all of you had a wonderful Thanksgiving – we are very thankful for our loving and supportive family and friends! – Linda

December 2, 2009 8:44 pm

Bennett developed a fever last night accompanied by body aches and chills so I took him back to the oncology unit this morning. They did blood tests (counts were good) and gave him fluids, more anti-nausea meds and some steroids. The oncologist also started him on antibiotics in case he's developing an infection (he was coughing a little but his chest X-ray looked good). This afternoon he was feeling much better (stopped for Chinese food and practiced for 30 minutes), but he'll go back to Winchester tomorrow for the same treatment. – Linda

December 4, 2009 5:12 pm

Today has been better. I managed to practice this morning and walked outside this afternoon – not my usual mile, but about half a mile. I'm still taking this one day at a time, knowing that each day is one day closer to being healthy again.

I look forward to your messages – even brief ones. Thanks for your love and prayers.

December 8, 2009 8:58 am

My near term goal has been to play the rehearsals and concerts this week with the Hagerstown Municipal Band. Well, I played a two hour rehearsal last night. The rehearsal was in Chambersburg, PA – about 1 ½ hours away. Linda drove me there because she wasn't sure I would be able to make the whole rehearsal. BUT I DID. I was exhausted by the end, but the goal I had set back in September has been met in spite of the setback of the second surgery and reaction to

the chemo last week. Lots of rest today and tomorrow, and I will be ready for the second rehearsal and
two concerts.

It was overwhelming to be sitting in the trumpet section with my musical friends. I had a hard time holding back tears at the end of the rehearsal, realizing that if it were not for the excellent medical people who work on my behalf, the caregivers here in Berkeley Springs, and the love and prayers of all my family and friends, I would not have reached what just a few short weeks ago seemed like an impossible dream. Thank you all for your continuing love and support. And thanks to the great conductor above who is clearly not ready to have me drop out of the trumpet section any time soon.

The most important person of all in this adventure continues to be my wife, Linda. Her untiring devotion and encouragement provide me with a window to the future and a pathway to getting there. Linda shares her fears and positive outlooks as they come with honesty and more love than anyone could imagine. We bolster each other when the need arises and celebrate the good moments as they come.

Without Linda, I could not possibly get through the challenges cancer and chemo present. Her spirit guides us and prevails.

December 11, 2009 9:08 am

Well, I made it through the second rehearsal last night. But I must admit that I am extremely tired this morning. The doctors are right about this intense level of chemo making me tired. Nevertheless, I am looking forward to playing the concert tonight. The conductor of the band has been very caring in asking Linda how I am doing. Julie and grandson Hunter are coming to the concert tonight and then will spend tomorrow with us.

Since Tuesday I have been losing my hair. Another prediction right on time. :-) That is all for now. It is 9:15 am and I need a nap.

December 12, 2009 2:54 pm

I MADE IT!!! The concert went very well. I was pleased with my playing as were my fellow section guys. I won't say it was easy, but I will say I feel good about reaching an important goal for me.

Thank you all for your love and prayers. Keep 'em coming 'cause they are working.

December 16, 2009 9:48 am

I had my second chemotherapy session yesterday – 5 hours 30 minutes. While there was some burning with the taxol (3 hours of this chemical), the nurse was able to fix it immediately. Yea!

They do blood work before going ahead with the treatment to determine if my hemoglobin is healthy enough to withstand the chemicals. Dr. Houck said my blood report was "boring," the word he uses to depict no problems. He also said he was pleased to see me back since he had told me to do the first treatment and decide if the effects were more than I wanted to deal with. He was also happy to hear I had done the rehearsals and concert (as were the oncology nurses who remembered I had talked about that as a goal.) He now knows that I am not a quitter.

Linda continues to be an amazing caregiver. Her concern and love are the major contributors to my pathway to being healthy. (from Linda – It's my husband who is amazing. His spirit and determination are indomitable. And with his almost bald head, he is getting sexier all the time!)

Linda bought me gift to celebrate my playing last week – an indoor putting green. She said now I can practice not only the trumpet, but my putting in anticipation of a return to golf this coming spring.

I feel your love and support surrounding me every day.

December 21, 2009 11:41 am

Today is day seven after my second chemo treatment and seems to be a little better than the days up to now, although I am as weak as a soaked noodle. Dr. Houck said he could give me Ritalin to boost my energy level, but I don't want to risk some of the possible side effects. I know this is all part of the journey and try to maintain a positive attitude towards it all, repeating the affirmation that now appears above all of my postings.

We had close to two feet of snow, and yesterday Linda went out and shoveled the walk and the decks. A guy came by and was able to plow out about a foot or so of the driveway snow, enough so Linda can get the Subaru in and out. The rest will have to wait for sunshine to melt it away. And maybe the sunshine will melt away the exhaustion I feel.

December 24, 2009 3:57 pm

I spent most of Tuesday and Wednesday in the oncology room at the hospital. Seems I am not tolerating the high dosage of chemo they have given me and for the second time needed to be given major fluids to gain any sense of well being. It seems to have worked, and I feel much better today. Dr. Houck said that beginning with my next treatment, my chemo schedule would be once every week for 3 weeks then a week off. If I am able to tolerate the reduced dosage, we will finish the chemo on that schedule.

Linda and I want to wish you all a very happy holiday. We wish you holidays bright and merry and a New Year filled with health, happiness and many blessings!

"Life is short and we do not have too much time to gladden the hearts of those who travel the way with us; so be swift to love and make haste to be kind; and may the blessing of the One who made us and who loves us and who travels with us be upon us, and remain with us always."

(A prayer from a Washington National Cathedral Community of Reconciliation service)

Thank you for traveling this journey with us.

Ending Chemotherapy

When you listen to your body, you become aware of just what you are capable of, and importantly, what alters the quality of your life to the degree that your body says "no more." I found an argument going on between my desire to do everything possible to go on living and my body telling me that to continue along the road I was on would destroy the quality of whatever life I might have left. I learned to listen to my body and to honor its messages.

All along in this journey I have been helped in listening to my body in all of its dimensions by people who possess special gifts in using spiritual energy in the healing process. The experiences I have had are undeniably powerful and intense. They have furthered my belief in the mysterious energy that connects all of us.

January 3, 2010 12:46 pm

I am wrestling with whether or not I will continue chemo. Dr. Houck is recommending a reduced dosage, which he thinks might make a difference in how my body handles the strong chemicals he is using. I am tempted to try this approach, but the truth is I am so tired and weak all the time that I just want it to all be over. I will probably start it and see if it is less harsh on my body and mind. Please pray for me to know what to do.

I am sorry to sound down, but this is just so hard.

January 5, 2010 3:31 pm

Well, dear family and friends, it turns out that Dr. Houck felt I looked a little weak to withstand a chemo treatment today. My blood work was all fine as were other vital signs, but he was not satisfied with how I looked. He said my "drawers were dragging." We have scheduled the smaller dosage treatment for next week. If that goes well, then we will do the next two consecutive weeks.

I asked him about the twitching I have at night, and he asked if I liked tonic water because quinine is good for that. I said "yes," and he said while I was at it, I should add a shot of vodka or gin. He said one drink a day would not interfere with the pain medicine I am now in the process of stopping.

So, cheers to all. I will try my best to get stronger. Dr. Houck did say there is no way to tell if continuing with the 1/3 dosage or stopping now makes any difference, but he was glad I said I would try to continue.

January 12, 2010 2:25 pm

I have gone for the first treatment at 1/3 the dosage. It took only 3 hours vs. 5 ½ for the full power blast. The oncology nurse said this should be much easier to tolerate. We will know in a day or two.

The extra days did have me feeling a little stronger. I was able to walk on the treadmill for 20 minutes each day starting Saturday, and I think I will be able to do that again today. Yesterday was a difficult day of decision making – wrestling with should I or should I not continue the treatments. I finally decided that if I did not try, I would not know if I could have completed the full regimen. Also, the person who has given me so much spiritual help through all of this – Linda – supported this approach and added she believed there was no more cancer to get rid of. She thought these additional treatments would be sort of a cleanup. Her words felt right to me.

The other news is that I am now in my third day being off of Vicodin, the narcotic I have been taking for pain. I spent two weeks reducing the dosages, and I think all is fine. My brain still feels a little fuzzy, but that could well be the chemo.

Sleeping has not been easy the past several nights, but now that the path forward has been determined and begun, it should be easier. Linda remains a blessing in my life; she is amazing at how she is coping with the stress of all of this. I know it is your love and prayers that are helping both of us.

January 16, 2010 3:18 pm

From Linda – Today is our 28th anniversary – how lucky we are to share this precious love and life together! Bennett asked that I write this update and tell it "like it is."

The 1/3 chemo dose has left him feeling far worse than the first two major doses – much vomiting from the chemo, more nausea meds and feeling somewhat better (we did get to go out for dinner to celebrate my birthday), then severe muscle twitches, dizziness, extreme fatigue, and balance problems. I took him to the oncology center, and our regular oncologist's father (also in the practice) thought that many of the problems were a side effect of the drugs he's taking to counteract the side effects of chemo. So Bennett stopped the nausea and the sleep medication. The twitching, etc. disappeared, but the acute nausea and debilitating fatigue have continued.

Before he took the 1/3 chemo dose, he had decided to give the chemo one more chance. Given that he's feeling horrible, has felt horrible for a long time, and wants to feel good again, he has decided to stop the chemo treatments. The last time we saw Dr. Houck, he said that whatever decision Bennett made would be a good decision given the very slight benefit of chemo in Bennett's particular case. And who knows, Bennett might have gotten that 5% benefit already.

We choose to see this decision as one that comes out of strength – the strength to move forward on this healing journey, foregoing chemo but embracing all of the life-enhancing options that are open to us. I know that all of you will hold him in your arms and keep him in your prayers as he sets out to regain his strength.

January 23, 2010 11:02 am

I thought I would share how things are going. The oncologist agreed with my decision to stop the chemo. His thinking was that as a preventive measure, any further gain that MIGHT be derived was not worth what I was going through, which was very bad. So as of today, I can report that each day has gotten a little better than the day before, and last night I actually got some real sleep for the first time in almost two weeks.

My improvement is a testament to the love and prayers I am so fortunate to receive from Linda and all of you. Don't stop now – it's working. :-)

January 31, 2010 11:31 am

In gratitude to all of you for your healing prayers and messages of love, I want you to know that I am definitely getting better and stronger. As of this past week I am practicing the trumpet again (15-20 minutes each day and practicing for longer periods every few days) and sleeping in 2-3 hour blocks and then falling asleep again. The weather has not been warm enough to walk outside, so I have "mapped out" a path in the house that I walk for 10-15 minutes continuously each day. Even my appetite is beginning to return. To use a baseball analogy, I am rounding 2nd and headed for 3rd. :-)

I love hearing from you. Your messages are a source of my returning energy.

February 8, 2010 1:14 pm

I continue to improve every day and am sleeping better each night. Yea!! I am practicing a little more each day as strength and endurance begin to improve. It does feel good to be playing again.

Again, thank you all for the love and prayers. They work!!!

February 14, 2010 2:04 pm

This has been a pretty good week. I feel a little stronger every day. If the nerve issues in my right hand and arm would get better faster, I would feel even better. The nerve damage was caused by the position they had my arm strapped in during both surgeries. I am working with a therapist who has experience with this type of injury as well as working with scar tissue. He is helping – I just get impatient.

Today, I pushed the trumpet practicing to an hour. My lung capacity is better, but still significantly reduced. So I just breathe more frequently. :-)

As I do better, Linda does better. We are both tired of the snow and the cold. We still have a lot of snow on the ground and more is predicted.

Happy Valentine's Day to all of you. Thank you all – the energy is so positive it is doing much for my healing.

February 21, 2010 11:58 am

Each day gets a little better. This week there has even been some improvement with my right hand/fingers and the range of motion of my right arm. The therapist says this is a slow process, but I am seeing small improvements each week. Yea!!

Not much improvement in my trumpet playing. I am having problems with dry lips that seem to limit what I can do. If any of my trumpet colleagues have any suggestions, I would be glad to hear them. I am using vitamin E at night as suggested by one player, but so far it hasn't helped much. I am sure it will get figured out and get better.

Love to all of you. Thanks so much for letting me know you are there.

March 1, 2010 11:22 am

I have never been more convinced that the cancer is gone from my body. This weekend I walked a lot – around a shopping mall looking for comfortable shoes one day and a mile outside with a friend the next.

My lip problem is improving. As a result of some research and the advice of some of my trumpet colleagues who read this page, I started using "CHOPSAVER." It is working very well. Yesterday, I played for about an hour and a half for the second time this week.

The therapist continues to "torture" me once a week and has really helped the nerve problem in my hand and the range of motion that was limited by the muscle relocation and surgical scars. I can now lift my right arm almost as high as my left. I will try a golf swing later this week.

The power of your love, thoughts and prayers continue to influence my improvement and Linda's well being. The better I get, the better she gets.

March 8, 2010 10:27 am (a day before my 72nd birthday)

I continue to improve, and I feel like I have rounded 3rd. My first public performance since ending chemotherapy was yesterday. Next: Easter Sunday, a concert with our Community Choir, Earth Day, and a wedding in May.

Now that the sun is beginning to shine, my walking has increased to 1.5 miles per day. The goal for this week is 2 miles per day. And I did hit golf balls in my friend Al's basement last Tuesday. It was OK – a little more restricted swing, but that is probably a good thing. I hope to do more
this week.

This coming Saturday we are driving to PA to see Julie and family. This will be my first "trip" since traveling to Charlottesville to see Dr. Kozower.

Both of us know that our recovery and health are because of the wall of love and prayer all of you have formed around us. Thank you and know that our love for you is heartfelt every day.

March 17, 2010 8:58 pm

I am doing OK – walking 1-1½ miles almost every day, and the trumpet practicing is fine.

The nerve issue in my right hand continues to improve, but it is still a problem. I try to ignore it, realizing that it may still be several months before the numbness is gone. The same is true for the numbness and feeling of a small animal sitting on my right side. Again, I know this will take lots of time before it feels somewhat normal.

I don't mean to sound like I am complaining – I am not – just letting all of you know what my real status is. This is a
long journey.

April 3, 2010 10:03 am

I wish you all a Happy Passover and Easter. Linda and I have much to celebrate – especially all of you – the loving people who have helped us through very trying times. We are so grateful for all of you.

I went to Beaufort, SC with Linda, and while she worked, I practiced the trumpet and played a little golf. The golf was OK with much room for improvement, but considering where I was six months ago, this is a miracle.

My recovery continues as the therapist works on me every week to stretch muscle and break up the scar tissue adhesions. The nerve damage to my right hand is healing slowly. It is now only a small nuisance when playing the trumpet.

No Cancer

Finding that cancer has left brings a sense of relief that cannot be described. As you will read, the news is not always wrapped in a pretty package, but good news is good news, period. Before getting to the good news, I was convinced that any and all new physical conditions were linked to cancer. Writing this more than two-and-a-half years later, I can attest that this shadow never goes away. Each report of good news simply confirms that survival from cancer is day to day.

April 8, 2010 9:12 am

I hardly know how to begin this update. The news is great, but how I got this news was more difficult.

This past week I had a brief episode of shortness of breath, and I was flushed and sweaty. The week before – after 10 days of somewhat mild abdominal pain – I went to the doctor and was diagnosed as having a stomach virus (much of that is going around). This most recent episode of shallow breathing caused Linda to take me back to the doctor who was very concerned that I was still having pain. He put me on oxygen and had me wheeled across the parking lot to the hospital for some blood work and a chest X-ray. The diagnosis was pneumonia, and he ordered me transferred to Winchester Medical Center where there is an excellent pulmonary unit with the capability of more extensive testing.

For three days I was examined every which way you can imagine, including a CT scan, ultrasound exams of all of my organs, blood cultures, an endoscopy and a colonoscopy. The results of all these tests were negative. THE CT SCAN SHOWED NO SIGNS OF ANY CANCER IN MY LUNGS; THE OTHER TESTS SHOWED NO SIGNS OF ANY CANCER ANYWHERE! AND NO PNEUMONIA! What looked like fluid on the X-ray was actually a shadow of the muscle that was pulled down during the second surgery to close the hole in my lung.

The bottom line is that they have no idea what is generating the pain. The internist at the hospital thinks it may well be muscular and/or skeletal caused by the healing from the surgeries. So I am home and back resuming my daily life, but with the relief that there is no evidence of cancer anywhere in my body.

Clearly the circle of prayers and love you have placed around Linda and me is very strong and is protecting me. As of this writing I am treating this mild pain as muscular. It didn't prevent me from playing well this past weekend, and I will refuse to let it interfere with the playing I will do in the future.

April 15, 2010 7:14 pm

Dr. Kozower has confirmed the results of the CT scan done in Winchester last week. All is clean – no problems. He emphasized that the first two years are critical to watch and so far – seven months into the two years – things look good. I am scheduled for another CT scan in July. Please do keep me in your thoughts and prayers. THEY ARE WORKING VERY WELL.

I played golf yesterday and am playing three times next week! I am overjoyed to be enjoying life again.

May 23, 2010 4:25 pm

I have not communicated in awhile as we have been away. We had a great train trip out west to see children, grandchildren and Linda's aunt and cousin. I did manage to practice the trumpet almost every day so I was ready to play a wedding gig when we got home. I've also been to New York to see Dr. Mathai, the holistic doctor I consulted shortly after the surgeries. The report from him is very good. He says my spirit and attitude are very positive and that makes a difference in the healing. He asked about my energy level, and I said it was about 80%. He felt this was normal and thought it would continue to improve. I just get impatient some days when I feel more tired than I want to be, but I must remind myself that it is seven months since the second big surgery and four months since the end of the chemo.

Thank you all for your continuing prayers and love. It is a huge part of my recovery. We are past the first critical seven months of the first critical two years. I take nothing for granted so stay by my side.

June 24, 2010 3:31 pm

I just heard from one of my friends that there has not been a CarePages message in a while. True. I am not ignoring you; I'm just busy getting stronger all the time. I would say that most days I am about 90% of my "normal" self, playing golf 3-4 times a week and rehearsing in Hagerstown on Monday and Thursday evenings with a concert every Sunday evening. I have also been doing a lot of grant writing for the county recycling program.

Whenever I get a little frustrated with my energy level, Linda reminds me that it was just eight months ago that I came home from the surgeries and five months ago that I stopped chemo. She thinks that my activity level is amazing, and I guess she is right. I don't know about amazing, but I do know that your prayers and love as well as my determination have led to good things. Thank you.

I hope you all are enjoying a good summer. It is very hot here this week, but you will never hear me complain. I wake up every morning looking down at the grass. How can you complain about that?

July 9, 2010 2:26 pm

The CT scan report is "No evidence of tumor recurrence or metastatic disease." Yea Team!!! And yes, you are my team. The acupuncturist I see said just yesterday that I am being protected by love and prayers coming from so many people that nothing could penetrate that shield. Linda and I thank you for being "our team" and love all of you.

September 5, 2010 12:27 pm

Sept. 9 will mark the first anniversary of my surgery, and I am celebrating my wellness. I have almost all of my energy back. Linda and I played in Julie's church in Bloomsburg (PA) last weekend to thank all of her fellow parishioners for their prayers. Wish we could play for all of you in thanks for your prayers.

By the way, I don't think I posted the latest PSA number: 0.29. The urologist was delighted. The prostate cancer procedure is now more than a year and a half ago.

The journey continues in bright sunshine.

November 9, 2010 7:37 pm

It has been two months since I last wrote. It has been an amazing time celebrating the one-year anniversary of so many difficult times now turned good. Every day Linda and I thank the universe for providing such caring people who have formed an incredible protective circle around us. I have no illusions as to why I am doing so well; it is the love and prayers given so caringly by all of you. Thank you from the bottom of my heart.

Here is how well you have done: yesterday I worked in the garden for four hours helping with the winterizing chores. Today I played golf, walking the front nine holes. This Sunday I am playing in

Linda's church, and later this month, I am playing two performances of "The Trumpet Shall Sound," the "Hallelujah Chorus" and a piece with the local children's choir in a community choir concert. In December I will play a concert with the local community band and a concert with the Hagerstown Municipal Band.

Last week I saw the holistic doctor that has helped me so much. He said I was doing really well and had a great spirit. Many thanks to all of you for keeping me here.

January 6, 2011 5:45 pm

YOU ARE ALL MEMBERS OF AN INCREDIBLE SUPPORT COMMUNITY!!! Linda and I have just returned from UVA in Charlottesville where I had my 16 month CT scan and visit with Dr. Kozower. His report: No signs of any inflammation in the lymph nodes or any thing else – all clear. He did say, with a huge smile, that there was a piece of my lung missing. I said that I thought he had a lot to do with that condition, along with my excellent health.

I played ten performances during November and December, thanks to the energy I receive all the time from your love and prayers. Please know how very much you all mean to us. You are all such a big part of my recovery. We love all of you for continuing to send such positive and caring energy.

June 19, 2011 10:50 am

As was said to the hangman, "No noose is good news." I have been enjoying good health and a high activity level since my last posting. I am working one day a week at the local golf course and playing three nights per week in Hagerstown, including a concert every Sunday evening. We are grateful for all of you and celebrate your caring with the dawn of every new day.

Cancer Returns

After almost two years of no cancer, the idea of being a survivor was transformed into the act of surviving. Survivor was a label to be applied to someone who is rid of something. Cancer demands that the individual enter into the ongoing act of surviving. Did I have – did we have – the strength to make yet further decisions about paths to survival? There is an expression that says you are never handed more than you are capable of handling. The months that followed would test us and the strength of our faith in our caregivers.

July 23, 2011 10:13 am

According to Dr. Houck, my CT scan "got my interest." He said there is a lymph node in the chest area that is 1.1 cm. Normal is 1 cm. After comparing this new CT scan with the one done in January, Dr. Kozower called me to say that he saw no significant difference. He said not to worry! Dr. Houck will do another CT scan in 3 months. I am thankful that I have just about made it – and will make it – through the first two critical post-operation years.

Soooo . . . Life goes on! Thanks for keeping me protected with all of your love and concern. Love and gratitude.

October 20, 2011 5:48 pm

My October CT shows that the lymph node that looked slightly enlarged in July has gotten somewhat larger. Dr. Houck has reviewed the CT scan with Dr. Kozower, and they want me to have a PET scan. While not urgent, it will get done within the next two weeks. While Dr. Houck talked about what the immediate next steps might be should the PET scan show that the node is "hot" (cancerous), both he and Dr. Kozower do not want to get ahead of the test results.

The fact that I have made it this far (25 months) is a good sign. I know that both Linda and I will deal with whatever the powers that be present to us. I have much life left to live and, as I said to Dr. Houck, a commitment to play at Dr. Kozower's son's Bar Mitzvah in August 2022.

So, keep the circle of light around me that your prayers and love have provided.

November 3, 2011 6:22 pm

As is frequently the case, the results of the PET scan are inconclusive. The next step will be a biopsy of three lymph nodes. The procedure will be done at UVA. Dr. Kozower is the one in charge, and I'll be talking with him tomorrow. Thank you for your caring.

November 8, 2011 5:37 pm

There is an expression that all things come in threes – good as well as not so good. The biopsy I had in Charlottesville today indicates that three lymph nodes located behind my trachea are cancerous. This is my third cancer challenge. The last two I have fought successfully and I will do the same with this challenge to balance what are now three bad things with three good fights.

When I saw Dr. Kozower yesterday, he indicated that he would not have set up the biopsy if, in the case of finding cancer, the cancer would not be treatable. While a surgical solution would not be practical because of the location of these enlarged nodes, there would be radiation and chemotherapy treatments available. I will see Dr. Houck and a radiologist in Winchester to learn about what is possible. Linda and I will then make an informed decision as to the next step.

On the plus side is that the growth of these three lymph nodes is very slow – a good thing. Also on the plus side is the impenetrable circle of love and prayer that all of you have surrounded me with for the past two+ years that I know you will continue to provide. Know that I have a lot more notes to play!

November 16, 2011 8:22 am

Our visits yesterday with Dr. Flax (radiation oncologist) and Dr. Houck were confrontations with the harsh realities of the alternatives available to deal with the recurrence of my lung cancer. At the outset, let me say that they both couched their recommendations in terms of preserving the quality of my life and extending the quantity of that life. These goals are critically linked; quality being the most important. Quantity without quality is certainly not what I want.

Dr. Flax has prescribed 35 radiation treatments (five per week for seven weeks). Both he, Dr. Houck and Dr. Kozower urge that I do chemotherapy with the radiation. It appears that chemotherapy weakens the cancer cells and almost doubles the effectiveness of the radiation. All of them dismiss a surgical solution for several reasons: surgery cannot address all of the lymph nodes that might now or potentially be involved, my body structure (scoliosis) would make any surgical attempt quite challenging and even less effective, the follow up to surgery would be radiation and chemotherapy, and surgery would require a significant recovery period leaving me in a weakened condition from which to undergo the follow up processes.

We discussed the scheduling of this combined treatment. I explained that I had several playing engagements over the next six weeks, playing that I have been looking forward to and really want to do. The response from Dr. Flax and Dr. Kozower was the same – these enlarged nodes appear to be very slow growing and delaying the treatments six weeks would not make much (if any) difference.

Dr. Houck acknowledged that he knew playing the trumpet is, indeed, a significant part of my quality of life. I should add that based on my difficult experience two years ago with chemotherapy, Dr. Houck will make an appropriate adjustment with the chemo regimen. He added that were I to have a reaction to chemo that was like my last experience, he would stop that part of the treatment and have me proceed with radiation alone.

None of this is without side effects, which I won't go into here. Suffice it to say that none involve increased body strength or the ability to play higher/louder/longer notes or hit longer drives.

At this point I am going in for the radiation mapping on December 6 with treatments planned to begin on December 27. Linda and I will also explore some other protocols that might have the potential of enhancing this plan.

Your caring, love and prayers have gotten Linda and me to this point of our lives, now more than two years distant from the first challenge. Please keep us close and dear as we continue on our journey.

December 20, 2011 7:48 am

I have received some homeopathic medicines from the holistic doctor I see a few times each year. These medications are to help me deal with the possible side effects of the treatments as well as to fight the cancer itself. In addition, I have been seeing a healer and am also following other protocols such as acupuncture, massage therapy and Reiki.

Together with the love and prayers that come from all of you, I know that soon I will be rid of this latest group of not-so-good cells.

Chemotherapy (Again) and Radiation

The cancer-free months strengthened me sufficiently to embark on the trail of surviving cancer yet another time. The love and healing energies sent to me on a daily basis from Linda, my family and friends fueled my determination to survive. Only for brief periods of time during the next months did I allow for not surviving. The support given to me on a daily basis from the nurses and technicians charged with administering what they knew to be necessary poisons into my body carried me through two months of treatments.

December 31, 2011 2:55 pm

Just a quick update to wish all of you a Happy New Year. I am somewhat uneven today – queasy and tired and then OK. This is to be expected after four radiation treatments and one chemo treatment. I am dealing with it, resting as needed and using ginger to control the queasiness in my attempt to avoid putting more drugs than necessary in my body. I am trying to maintain a program of exercise and practicing (trumpet) interspersed with rest. Linda will do Reiki again today, and I am meditating every day.

It is very helpful knowing that all of you are keeping me in your thoughts and prayers.

January 22, 2012 1:49 pm

I have now completed seventeen radiation and four chemotherapy treatments. I am halfway through this regimen and happy to report that the negative effects have been minimal. There have been a few moments of queasiness on just a few days. Fatigue sets in most afternoons, but I continue to eat well. The chemo nurses are amazed and think that there are a few factors at work: I drink about 2-3 liters of water a day, I walk almost two miles every day (treadmill), I play the trumpet almost every day for about an hour, and I have a very positive attitude about the outcome of these treatments. The radiation people are surprised that I have no skin, breathing or swallowing problems. And I still have all my hair.

What the health professionals do not include in their assessment is the amazing circle of prayer, love and light provided by my friends and relatives that is protecting me. I know that you are there – all of you – all of the time.

February 14, 2012 1:14 pm

There is just one more radiation treatment left – tomorrow morning. Yea!!! I am writing today because many of you have inquired about how I am doing. In truth, this past week has not been much fun. I began to experience some side effects related to the radiation treatments last week, which at first were not too bad. Recently they have been getting progressively more intense. In addition to feeling tired in the afternoons, the side effect that was really tough was much pain when swallowing. The doctor explained that it was a burn in my esophagus, just like the burns on my chest area from the radiation. While there are ointments that can be applied to the skin, there is no such relief for the wall of the esophagus. Dr. Flax gave me some pain medicine (Tylenol with Codeine), which did make it a little more tolerable, but still, every time I swallowed – even my own saliva – it felt like there was a golf ball in my throat. OUCH!!!

By Sunday all I could do was force myself to eat soft food – force – because even that hurt with every swallow. And I could not drink much water because of the pain. By Monday I was dehydrated when Linda took me to my 33rd radiation treatment (33 of the scheduled 35). I was also very short of breath, so Dr. Flax ordered a chest X-ray to rule out pneumonia. No pneumonia! He then prescribed some stronger pain meds and ordered fluids by infusion. That was yesterday.

Today I am doing much better. I did celebrate Valentine's Day with treatment #34. The pain meds are helping mask the pain when I swallow, allowing me to drink plenty of water again. Dr. Flax explained that it might be a few weeks before the healing process completely takes care of the "golf ball" in my throat.

While pretty painful, this seems to be the only negative side effect I have experienced from either the radiation or the chemotherapy. Up until this past Saturday, I was walking two miles every day and playing the trumpet almost every day. I am planning on walking again today. The trumpet playing will have to wait until I am less "loopy" from the hydrocodone. (Too much concentration required.)

Thanks to all of you for your love and healing energy. All the bad stuff is almost gone, including, thanks to all of you and the circle of light and love you are providing, the cancer.

February 25, 2012 11:32 am

From Linda – We've hit a bump in the road, but Bennett is determined to get over it, around it, and through it. I brought him to the ER on Tuesday evening, and he's still in the hospital. His body is fighting – shivering (rigors), sweats, shortness of breath and weakness – everything that he would have with an infection except fever. And his white blood cell count is declining. They are testing for every kind of infection they can think of, but so far, all of the cultures are coming back negative. The doctor is giving him antibiotics in case it is an infection and Demerol to control the shaking.

Yesterday he had a CT scan, and there is good news – no signs of cancer! So your prayers, healing energy and love along with the chemo and radiation have accomplished what we hoped they would. Now if we can just conquer whatever is going on in his body.

Today we decided that perhaps his body worked so hard during the chemo/radiation treatments and subsequent narcotic medications for the esophageal burn that it's just been overloaded. This morning instead of staying in bed, Bennett got up, had breakfast, shaved, cleaned up and went for a short walk. In his words, "I've had enough of this s--t!" He's going to honor his body's need for reassurance and rest, but at the same time, he's going to try to get back to "normal" and not give in to worry and fear. In other words, he's going to get back to "give 'em hell, Bennett."

Send him strength and determination, love and prayers. And thanks for all of the powerful healing that you have sent already!

February 27, 2012 1:26 pm

It is official from Dr. Houck: "The result of the therapies [chemo & radiation] is EXCELLENT. The lymph nodes have been reduced to within normal limits and there is no sign of cancer anywhere." He thinks that my immune system fell following all of the treatments and is now making a comeback. He released me from the hospital, and I am to resume my normal schedule of activities as tolerated.

There is so much to be thankful for, not the least of which is the energies all of you have sent to me. It is with tears of joy in my heart that I send this message with great love.

Lingering Pain

We went on a train trip out to the west coast to see our family and to just plain relax after the recent battle. As you will read, I began to have some pain issues which I was convinced were related to cancer. I became somewhat depressed about this and did not talk about it with Linda for months. In fact, the only people I shared my concern with were the people in my Berkeley Springs cancer support group. It was the only time throughout this entire journey that I retreated inside myself and would not share my feelings with anyone other than members of my support group. It was a lonely time.

June 21, 2012 2:30 pm

I know it has been awhile since I last updated you on my health. Thanks to the many who have sent inquiries. I did not want to concern anyone with the problems I have been having for what is now about 2½ months. After my experiences over the past week, I can confidently say that I am in no danger from what I am about to describe – just some pain.

About mid-March after returning from our train trip out west, I began to have pain in the center of my upper abdomen and shortness of breath. I did not worry a whole lot about it, thinking it was probably some form of stomach flu. The conditions did not let up and finally, at the end of May, Linda got me to go to our family doctor. He thought it might be an ulcer and prescribed medication that I took for two weeks. There was no appreciable change so the meds were terminated. He did consult with Dr. Houck, and they ordered some blood work and an X-ray. Result: no cancer or anything out of the ordinary.

This week the pain was up to about a 7 and the shortness of breath was getting worse. So, back to my family doctor I went. Again, he consulted with Dr. Houck and then sent me to the local hospital for more tests: electrocardiogram, blood cultures and an ultrasound of my abdomen (gall bladder, pancreas, liver, etc). All tests came back negative.

Before doing an endoscopy, both doctors feel we should try an increase in the ulcer medication, which would also address any swelling that might be present in the connection between the stomach and duodenum. So that is what I am going to do for the next week. I do have a scheduled CT scan in July. It will be increased to cover the abdomen area. Both doctors agree that they would like to avoid, if possible, the invasiveness of an endoscopy.

I should add that through all of this I have managed to play all of the rehearsals and concerts of the Hagerstown Band, a performance with an organist on Mother's Day, golf once or twice each week, and work one day a week at the golf course.

I will let you know how this resolves. At least we now know it is not life threatening – and that is a good thing.

July 16, 2012 4:48 pm

I have just returned from seeing Dr. Houck and the results of the CT scan last week are "totally boring." There is no sign of any cancer anywhere. That is the really good news. The CT scan also did not show any irregularities anywhere that would cause the pain I am having. He thinks that it might be a spasm of the esophageal muscle and has ordered an endoscopy to have a look, although he says there is only a 5% chance that it might show something. In the meantime, he recommends quinine water – with or without the gin. (He smiled indicating that it would probably be better with the gin.)

Dr. Houck and my family physician think that the usual medications for this type of spasm – heart medications – would cause more problems than they might cure. They also think that if it is a spasm, it might just decide to quit at some point.

I am carrying on my usual activities. The pain comes and goes, but at least we are comforted by knowing there is no cancer, tumor or any other malfunctioning organ. YEA!!!

August 5, 2012 5:16 pm

As my cousin Rita has said, she doesn't know why these are called the golden years. They should be called the silver years because there is always something that is tarnished. I am beginning to feel like our parents when they got older – one doctor appointment after another.

I begin with the good news. Saw my urologist for my six month checkup. My PSA is now less than 0.1, so I have now been moved to an annual checkup schedule. Looks like the prostate cancer is a thing of the past.

Now for the saga related to the pain across my upper abdomen, which is still there. I have followed Dr. Houck's orders to drink quinine water (with gin), and I had an endoscopy that revealed nothing – all is normal. The doctor who performed the procedure seemed to think the pain might be caused by scarring from the radiation and chemotherapy treatments. Nothing to do about that except go on some pain medication. I am not interested in that remedy. Too many side effects.

Following the endoscopy, I saw my cardiologist, Dr. Kahn, for my annual checkup. (See what I mean by all the doctor appointments?) The cardiogram I had in his office showed some blockage in my right ventricle, which was verified during his exam.

He said it was not uncommon to have some damage following radiation to the area that was treated for the cancer. He also indicated that this type of damage could cause pain where I am experiencing it as well as the shortness of breath. So . . . good news: cancer gone; bad news: some side effects of scarring and damage to the heart – maybe. Next we scheduled a nuclear stress test. (I must say that the cardiologist's explanation about shortness of breath seems to fit with the fact that when I play the trumpet I am bringing more oxygen into my body. The same is true when I am play golf – exercising – and there is no pain. Maybe the treatment is more trumpet playing and more golf. :-)

The stress test showed that my heart is fine. What's next? Dr. Kahn referred me to a pain management unit in Winchester.

September 13, 2012 8:07 pm

After almost six months of pain and numerous tests and guesses by all of my doctors, it appears that Dr. Whitesitt (better known as my wife, Linda) may have hit the diagnosis on the button – costochondritis – an inflammation of the cartilage that connects the ribs to the breastbone. This diagnosis was confirmed by the pain management physician's assistant I saw today. She has prescribed a steroid treatment (oral), which I will begin tomorrow morning. If that does not prove completely effective, I will then have some steroid injections. She reviewed all of the test results and after declaring that I was incredibly healthy concluded that Linda's search of Mayo Clinic postings had revealed the answer. She also said that this was not an unusual side effect of radiation treatments to that area of the body. I hope you will join us in praying that we have a solution. Finally!

September 29, 2012 11:38 am

Plan A – the oral steroid pack did not work. I saw the pain management folks yesterday, and they went to Plan B – an injection of cortisone directly into the center of my chest bone. I should get relief within three to five days. If not, they will come up with a Plan C. They are very nice people and are trying hard to relieve me of the pain I have. Their diagnosis remains costochondritis.

I am off to Radford (VA) on Monday to guest conduct the University Wind Symphony and to be the guest lecturer in a few classes. I am looking forward to a fun week – hopefully pain free.

October 22, 2012 4:23 pm

I saw Dr. Houck today – "A boring CT scan report." No cancer anywhere, and all else looked fine. Regarding the pain – the steroid injection has helped, but there is still some pain. I see the pain doctor again in November. Perhaps I might need another injection or two. We will see.

You are all part of an incredible support team that has enormous powers at keeping me here.

Our Journey Continues

The pain in my chest finally subsided, and I didn't need any additional injections when I saw the pain management doctor's physician assistant in November and December 2012. That's the good news. The bad news is that my periodic three-month CT scan in mid-January 2013 indicated a troublesome mass in my right lung. Although we've been down this road before, when it comes to a possible diagnosis of cancer recurrence, experience doesn't make the path any easier.

January 24, 2013 4:39 pm

We have just returned from Dr. Houck's office where we received the report of the CT scan. His words – "half boring." There is a developing soft tissue density mass in my right lung. The radiologist calls it highly suspicious, but Dr. Houck feels it may well be caused by some kind of lingering respiratory infection for which I was treated almost three weeks ago. Dr. Houck has talked with Dr. Kozower and neither of them feels there is any cause for panic, but they want me to have a PET scan as soon as possible to see if this "mass" is "hot." If it is not, then this is a respiratory infection. If it is "hot," then they will want to biopsy it because "hot" readings on a PET scan are not conclusive. Once again, we are taking this one step at a time and not jumping to any conclusions.

This is not quite the New Years greeting I had hoped to deliver. Hopefully the next report will be fine. In the meantime, I keep all of you in my protective circle. If you have a minute, you might just crank up a little healing and spiritual energy and send it our way. As one of my supporters says, we will "keep on keeping on."

January 30, 2013 6:07 pm

I had the PET scan this morning and also a checkup this afternoon with Dr. Lessar, my pulmonary doctor. He did a breath test to determine current capacities which, as expected, have diminished since 2009 due mostly to surgery and radiation treatments. He also had the results of the PET scan. Suffice it to say, the report is not what we had hoped for. The soft mass had a high reading, and there is a lymph node below the mass that is just past what is considered acceptable. Dr. Lessar did say that the mass looks unusual and still might be something other than a malignancy. He knows that the next step is a biopsy, which after talking with Dr. Kozower, they decided to do at UVA.

Linda and I are both feeling that this is somewhat surreal. We have been here before and know that we will handle whatever it is. We continue to have complete faith in our medical team and know that Dr. Kozower will guide the actions he feels will produce the best outcome.

We are survivors! But the landmarks in this journey where survival has been thought possible were places where we knew what we were facing. It is in the territory of not knowing where thinking about survival seems almost impossible. During these days we vacillate between desperately wanting to hear that all of the tests have falsely pointed towards a recurrence of cancer and dreading that the news will portend more days when survival has to be fought and won every step of the way. It is all we can do to keep from simply clinging to one another in retreat. We know that for us quality of life will always trump quantity, and so we make the best of this difficult period, going about our usual activities with a minimum of cloudiness. We know that the path will soon be clear, and we plan to continue on this journey for some time to come. In the meantime, make no mistake about it — this is hard!

February 16, 2013 4:34 pm

Just got the biopsy report - - **NO CANCER!!!!** The small mass is scar tissue. That is what is causing the shortness of breath. Dr. K recommends that the next CT scan be done in 6 months. Let's all have a drink together and lift our glasses to life, love and each other. We love all of you. Bennett & Linda

There are no words to express the emotions we felt as the words "NO CANCER" began to wash over us. The Refuah Shelma (ancient Hebrew prayer for full healing) offered by so many friends, the healing energy transmitted by "Red" who ended our brief session by confidently announcing "it has been taken care of," and the circle of protection maintained by all those who continue to send love, prayers and positive energies have made possible the dawns of many more todays.

Experience has taught us not to question the how or why of any of it, simply to be thankful. Whatever the future holds, we pray that our journey goes on and on – at least until Dr. Kozower's son's Bar Mitzvah and our grandchildren's weddings! But however long our journey lasts, we will travel hand in hand with the love and support of our family and friends knowing that for now – for today – we are surviving cancer.

LINDA'S STORY

I tell my story about our surviving cancer journey in a chronological series of reflections that I began to write shortly before Bennett's lung cancer recurred in fall 2011. The reflections are in sets of four with each reflection in each set inspired by a word that begins with a letter in the word "life." For example, the first set of reflections were inspired by the words *L*ove, *I*nhale Exhale, *F*ear and *E*ndure. Meditating on words starting with the letters L-I-F-E gave me a structure for exploring my responses to living with Bennett's cancer, made it possible for me to give voice to my experiences during this exceedingly difficult and challenging journey, and kept me connected to LIFE.

Our journey is one with many colors. The metaphor of a colorful rainbow has lit the way in our relationship for more than thirty years ever since we heard Harry Chapin sing "Flowers are Red" in New York in 1980. From that moment on, we have been inspired by the idea that both life and our marriage need to embrace all the colors in the rainbow. Bennett frequently gives me a bouquet of many-colored carnations on special occasions as a reminder that in our life together, we vowed long ago to honor all the colors. The light times are easy; the dark ones are not. But we have survived many dark times before, and now we are surviving the darkest one of all. My story is an attempt to paint in words the rainbow of our surviving.

Reflection #1 (fall/winter 2011)

*L*ove

My husband and I are both classical musicians. I play the violin and viola, and Bennett is a conductor and trumpet player. Over the years we have come to know the old truth that music happens in the space between the notes. It is the mystery that rests between the notes as well as the nature of how they are connected that brings the notes on the page to life. It has been our goal to shape the relationship between the notes in such a way that we create music that moves us and the listener. The spaces and what they contain give the music meaning.

In the same way, the mystery that rests in the space between the moments of our life together flows through our relationship like a river and sustains us. For us, that mystery is love. Perhaps it's the same for music.

As we have moved through time together, the experience of that "time together" – the accumulation of all of the moments and the love between them – has carved out a shared history similar to how the unfolding in time of notes and spaces creates a memory of a unified work of art. Looking back, we see a musical work – and our marriage – as whole and indivisible, and neither one of us has been willing to tear it up and throw it away during the real hard times when we thought love had ceased to fill up the spaces. The wholeness and indivisibility of our shared life has always pulled us back. It is what remains with us just like the music is still present after the last note is played.

Love is what kept Bennett going before emergency surgery to repair a leak in the remaining portion of his right lung only a few weeks after his initial surgery for lung cancer in October 2009. Some time in the middle of the night before the early morning surgery, my husband's roommate, on hearing Bennett distraught and tearful, managed to move his bed close to Bennett's so that he could hold my husband's hand and pray with him. Bennett's roommate was not capable of getting out of bed, so we never have been able to figure out how he moved his hospital bed. But somehow he did, and in those terrifying moments late at night, he filled the space between them with love, assurance and comfort.

Bennett also shares a special relationship with someone else – his surgeon. We both know that his doctor's caring attention, his supportive communication and his commitment have helped lengthen the time in which we can both say, "We're surviving cancer." This is another space – the space between doctor and patient – that has been filled with love. And we know that relationships filled with love are healing.

Inhale Exhale

Sometimes the spaces between notes are filled with moments of silence – moments when players stop playing and singers stop singing. Many times these rests are moments for breaths between phrases. They form a container for the phrases they enclose. Music played without attention given to breathing between phrases is lifeless, without flow and without direction. Music, like life, needs breath to come alive.

There are many times in our journey of surviving cancer when breathing has eluded me. So many events have taken my breath away: sitting in the doctor's office and listening to him explain that the results of the biopsy showed cancer and, two years later, hearing that the cancer had returned; trying to take in another doctor's description of the side effects of chemotherapy and radiation; hearing the surgeon say that because he had found cancer in a lymph node outside of my husband's lung, it was Stage III cancer and not Stage I; answering a call from my husband and hearing him gasp that he couldn't breath. There have even been whole periods of time, days even, when it seemed like I couldn't breathe: the ten minutes it took me to get home not knowing if Bennett would still be breathing when I got there; the next two minutes waiting for the ambulance; the three hours driving behind the ambulance from our regional hospital to the hospital in Charlottesville; the days waiting for the results of CT and PET scans; the hours spent by Bennett's side while chemicals flowed into his body; the days between treatments as I watched his body become weaker and weaker.

When my husband started to heal after the surgery and chemotherapy, there were many moments when I felt I couldn't get my breath. Every time Bennett coughed, every time he sighed or groaned, my body would immediately shift into panic mode. Once when he yelled in frustration at some computer glitch, I was in tears by the time I got to the top of the stairs to see what the problem was. I drove my husband crazy with my constant query, "What's wrong?"

It was during those trying days of panic for no good reason that a wise friend gave me words, stories and strategies to help me make my way out of instant fright over every sneeze and cough. One of the things she suggested was to breathe – inhale and exhale deeply. She even gave me different breathing responses for different situations.

When I remember to breathe, the cancer doesn't go away. But just like the rests in music that form a container for musical phrases, my breath forms a container for the moments of my life, and I am reminded that for this moment, we are together. With each breath, I am thankful for the time we share. Breathing helps me feel connected to the life that surrounds me – my husband's breath, the rain on the window, the flowers in the path, and our cats asleep on the sofa. Breathing gives me the strength to rest in the moment no matter what it holds.

Fear

Fear is a frequent companion. I fear my husband dying. I fear what might happen to Bennett's body during chemo and radiation. I fear that the cancer will not respond to treatment. Now that the cancer has recurred (fall 2011), fear seems to be a constant, unwelcome, companion. It's a hollow pit in my stomach that won't go away.

Fear doesn't always visit with the same intensity. It comes in waves similar to the waves of grief I experienced after my mother's death. Sometimes, the strength of the wave knocks me off my feet. During the months when the CT scans showed nothing to worry about, the fear receded. But it always shows itself quickly when Bennett experiences a pain or a cough we can't explain. When Bennett is away in the evening for a rehearsal and I am in the house alone, a wave of fear can pull me under. The thought – "This is how it's going to be when he's gone" – washes over me. It isn't so much a matter of "I'll be alone." Instead, it's "How will I be able to go on when the 'I' that I am feels so intimately tied to the 'we' that we are?"

This is the source of the pit in my stomach in this journey of "we're surviving cancer." The ground beneath my feet is always shifting, and these earthquakes make me lose sight of who I am because my "I" is a "we." Who is the "I" in the "we're surviving cancer" story? It's not the same "I" as before there was any cancer. Confronted with the fragility of life, I want to hang on to how it was before cancer, and frankly, there are times that I get mad as hell that cancer has changed everything.

There was a time in the winter of 2010 during the "no signs of cancer" months when I found myself inexplicably angry at Bennett. It took me weeks to realize that being angry at him masked the horrible fear that it might be our last Christmas together. Once I discovered its source, my anger vanished, and with it, my fear.

Now it's another Christmas (2011), and the cancer is back. There is no anger this time, only fear. What helps? Writing these reflections is a comfort. Finding the words to describe what I have kept and continue to keep inside shines sunlight into dark and fearful places. Taking to heart the one very important word in the title of our book – "today" – helps abate my fear.

Today – this day – this moment – my husband and I are eating breakfast together, paying the bills together, having dinner with friends together. We're making music together, and he's helping me with my work. The "I" I am today is this woman who loves this man, who reaches out and touches him and leans over and kisses his cheek. Today we are both alive.

I have today with Bennett. I'd be lying if I said that it's enough.

Endure

It is in the small, sometimes inconsequential moments of our life together that I am frequently struck with the sudden, strong desire that "we" must endure. Fixing dinner, opening the mail, grocery shopping – these are some of the shared moments when I long that the pleasure of doing them together lasts as long as possible. In some ways, it's the same as holding onto glorious moments in classical music.

A few weeks ago the music ensemble that I direct and play in performed an arrangement of the "Nimrod" variation from Edward Elgar's *Enigma Variations*, a sublimely beautiful work. Playing it, I was deeply aware of every note, and many of them I held as if I didn't want to let them go. I savored each note's significance thoroughly before going on to the next. This practice of awareness is what I want to bring to every moment of our life together.

Cancer forces me to bring all of my awareness to the times my husband and I share. It also nudges me to be a more engaged witness in other encounters I have throughout the day. When I do, when I bring my awareness to the mountains before my eyes, the friend who is telling me about her day, the hummingbird's wings I hear as she flies above the feeder, the shiny rock that catches my attention, I find that my life fills with meaning. The moment endures. It is luminous.

I remember entering a busy airport after a weeklong spiritual retreat in an idyllic country setting. I was stunned. My time away had made me intensely aware of the radiance of every person I saw. It was as if every individual was lit from within – everyone special, everyone shining in this great web of life. The moment didn't last long, and I've never been able to recapture the depth of that experience, but my husband's cancer brings me close.

At this moment one of our cats jumped into my lap as I was writing these words. Instead of brushing him away, I paused, took him into my arms for as long as he allowed me to hold him, and became aware of the preciousness of this moment. He's not one to cuddle, so I had to treasure being with him fully and quickly. I want all of the moments in my life to endure, but my cat and life have other plans.

It occurs to me that "endure" has another meaning. Bennett is my hero when it comes to enduring many bouts with cancer without giving in to fear or pain. He has remained positive and optimistic throughout the surgeries and the chemo and is refusing to yield to despair when faced with lung cancer recurrence and the prospect of radiation and more chemo. In all of the health updates to family and friends he has written, there has never been even a hint of anger or despondency.

I have never known my husband to be anything but hopeful and determined. It is his indomitable will that has carried both of us through the sometimes bumpy terrain of our life together. It is his unwavering commitment to me and to life that lifts me up in the moments when I lose heart. His words also help – "No matter what happens, Linda, we will endure."

I want us to endure. Bennett teaches me how.

Reflection #2 (fall/winter 2011)

Let Go

I direct a small ensemble comprised of amateur and professional musicians. One of the things I help them work on is how to release the sound at the end of notes. How one lets go of a note, how one connects the end of one event with the beginning of another, and how one stops the sound but lets the memory of the sound continue are important in creating flow, direction and energy in music.

I am fairly successful teaching my musician friends how to let go; I'm not successful instructing my heart how to let go of the moments I share with my husband. I try to practice Buddhist non-attachment, but I admit to being really attached to all of the moments we have together. Perhaps it's my sentimental nature.

Years ago my thesis advisor wrote in red ink all over my answer to a question on an application for a fellowship, "Don't you think you're being naïve and sentimental here." I interpreted her pejorative "sentimental" as meaning shallow and somewhat self-indulgent, maybe even nostalgic. Perhaps I read too much into her comment, but I was devastated.

Today I'm much more sure of myself, and I find I have no trouble wearing the mantle of someone who is "sentimental" – someone who is influenced by emotion rather than reason or fact. That definition fits my inability to let go of our treasured moments to a "T." No amount of reason or fact encourages me to let go of them.

What does help me let go of these moments is how I let go of musical sounds. I can't hang on to them forever or else the music stops. The passage of time simply makes it impossible for me to hold on to them. I have to make a choice how to let them go. I end notes with grace, give attention to how they connect with the notes that follow and, at the end of the composition, I release the last note and imagine its sound reaching toward the horizon. Then I look back and hear in my mind's ear how all of the moments of "letting go" have shaped a singular performance of black notes on a white page.

In our life together I can do no less. Playing music teaches me that I must fill our moments' endings with beauty, attend to the ones that come next and, at the end of our life together, know that what we have shared will extend beyond what I can see, but not beyond what I can feel and remember.

"*I*mpulse of Will"

In her book *The Modern Conductor*,[1] Elizabeth Green describes "impulse of will" – the ability to *will* a musical event to happen – as a vital quality in a conductor. Bennett has an amazingly strong "impulse of will" as a conductor and as a person who survives cancer day after day. I will always remember a comment made by one of my husband's colleagues after Bennett had finished conducting a university band concert. The colleague was surprised by how wonderful the band sounded because he knew that many students in the band had to struggle to play their instruments. "They had no right to sound that good!" he quipped. But they did; they had Bennett to lead them. He has always had the "impulse of will" and the technique to help band and orchestra members play better than they thought they could. He wills it to happen.

In the same way, Bennett willed our marriage to happen and has willed it to survive. He wooed me with such a strong sense of will that I had no alternative but to say "yes" to his proposal. When we were going through a rocky stretch and I thought that stepping out of the marriage might be easier than staying in it, he refused to give up

---

[1] 2nd ed. Englewood Cliffs, NJ: Prentice-Hall, Inc., 1969, p. 14.

on us and willed us together again. I see the same powerful will in his encounter with multiple cancers.

Over and over again I have observed that Bennett wills his body to do more than I think he can do. In December 2009, less than two months after his second lung cancer surgery – a surgery which had come close on the heels of his first – and during the weeks he was undergoing grueling chemotherapy, he became determined that he was going to play in a municipal band Christmas concert. I watched every morning as he stretched his right arm up the shower stall trying to regain his range of motion. He could barely get it high enough to hold the trumpet. I knew that Bennett was so tired that he could hardly sit up for more than half an hour or so. How on earth was he going to sit through a two-hour rehearsal, not to mention blow into a trumpet for two hours? But Bennett is nothing if not determined. I drove him the hour it took to get to the rehearsal, asked his stand partner to keep an eye on him, and then sat in the auditorium fully expecting that after half an hour or so I would have to help him into the car and take him home.

I had forgotten Bennett's "impulse of will." He not only made it through the rehearsal, but also the next one a few days later, and the concert at the end of the week. I have never been so thankful for the strength of his determination. It was a wonderful Christmas present for both of us.

There have been several occasions when my husband's will has faltered. The most difficult aspects of chemotherapy were the side effects, not just from the chemo, but also from the drugs that he took to counteract those side effects. There were numerous debilitating physical side effects, but the emotional ones were also painful. The drugs robbed Bennett of his willpower. They took away his "Bennett-ness." I think it was when that happened that he decided that he had had enough. A little more than half way through the treatments (early 2010), he stopped them. Gradually his body and his will regained their strength. He returned to playing trumpet full-time during the summer months that followed and has continued to play to this day.

Bennett's determination is clearly evident in many of the email messages he has sent to friends during his surviving cancer journey. They give insight into his phenomenal ability to see the best in every situation, and it is this gift that is at the root of his "impulse of will." His faith in what his students were truly capable of, his tenacity and encouragement to help them work to uncover their potential, and his vision of what they could sound like as an ensemble drove the rehearsal process and lead to results that belied belief. In the same way, it is Bennett's unflinching determination to survive cancer for many days and years to come that fuels his life. He has a deep, deep desire to survive, and he is committed to willing that to happen.

Figuring It Out

Neither Bennett nor I like dallying. We look at a situation, digest information regarding what needs to be done, make decisions fairly quickly about what to do, and then do it. We waste little time chewing on problems. Surviving cancer throws a monkey wrench into our "standard operating procedure."

While Bennett was recuperating at home after his lung cancer surgeries and during those weeks I was trying to process the news that what doctors had thought was stage I cancer was actually stage III, I spent days on the computer reading about cancer and chemotherapy. I also gathered as many books and pamphlets on how to keep cancer from recurring as I could. I became obsessed with "figuring it out." If I read just one more study, one more article, I would find the answers I needed. I wanted to know what Bennett should do, what he should eat, what he should drink, and what alternative healing modalities he should try in order to make sure that the cancer never returned. I wanted answers. I wanted guarantees.

Well-meaning friends fed my obsession. "You need to have Bennett practice this technique, try this remedy, juice this beverage, listen to this healer, take these herbs." It seemed like their well-meaning advice was endless. I felt that if I listened to them, if I figured out what we should do, I could make sure that everything would be OK. With so much information and so much heart-felt advice, I knew I could figure out the answers and everything would get back to normal. I just knew it. I was driving myself, and Bennett, crazy.

As the effects of the chemo wore off and the circumstances seemed a little less desperate, I started to breath again, and Bennett and I were able to return to "figuring it out" together. We work much better as a team than I do "flying solo."

First, we decided that whatever we did, life was never going to get back to "normal." What would our "new normal" look like? We didn't know. We couldn't predict the next second let alone the future. The only thing we could be sure of was the moment we were in right then. With that realization came the conviction that we had to concentrate on living where we were and not where we hoped we would be some day down the road. I had to stop worrying about "what if this is our last Christmas, our last trip together, our last anniversary," take a breath, and focus on the joy of having my husband at my side right now.

I also had to stop feeding my addiction for finding the right answers. We knew I would drive both of us batty trying to come up with just the right diet, the right drinks, the right supplements, and the right alternative therapies to ensure that the cancer did not return. I had to come to grips with the fact that there are no guarantees. What we decided to aim for was balance – eat healthy, organic, unprocessed food and, occasionally, some that might not be so healthy but that add to the quality of our life. (Bennett's occasional bagel with lox spread gives him immeasurable joy.) As for supplements and alternative healing modalities, we make our best guess based on research, intuition, and what Bennett's body is telling him.

In making the decision that we couldn't possibly do or eat or drink everything that was recommended in order to prevent cancer recurrence, we vowed we wouldn't go back and second guess ourselves. There would be no "if only we had done . . . " if the cancer came back. Now that the cancer has recurred, we're sticking to that resolution. We will continue to eat healthy meals and add those things that we feel augment the quality of our lives. It's come down to figuring out a balance that works for us.

*E*njoy

There is an art to finding balance in a musical ensemble. Too much of one line or instrument detracts from the whole. When I coach a string quartet, I must balance the group's sound by listening carefully to every player's part and make decisions regarding who should be prominent, who needs to support, and who needs to fill out the texture. When I cook, I create a tasty dish by paying attention to what flavors need to dominate, how much they should stand out, and the degree to which all of the other flavors need to be present in order to subtly add to the desired result.

Balancing one's life is also an art requiring close attention and careful listening. I find it particularly difficult when a loved one is surviving cancer, and I know that it's been a challenge for Bennett as well. The decisions that my husband has had to make concerning treatment options have required that he consider balancing the quality with the quantity of his life. For my part, I've had to struggle with how to balance the tremendous weight of my concern for Bennett with my equally strong desire to enjoy every moment of the time we have together. If I tip the scale in favor of my worry, I miss what's happening right now. If I lean too much in the direction of ignoring my fears and rest solely in "be here now," I feel like I cut out too much of my heart and that leaves me feeling empty.

Looking at myself over the last couple of years, I know that I err much more frequently on the side of worry – much more. So knowing myself, I realize that finding balance means that I add more enjoyment in my life. When I do that, I'm happier, and I know Bennett is.

A friend recently asked me, "What are you doing for yourself?" After I stumbled and stuttered for a while, she remarked that it was taking me far too long to answer her question. Later I realized that it's not that I don't do things for myself, it's just that I often don't think of the things I do for myself as "things I do for myself." Answering her question requires that I pay closer attention, just like I pay attention to balancing music and meals. It also requires that I pay attention to the "enjoyment" part of the things I do for myself – savor the moments so I really do enjoy them.

There is much in my life that I enjoy doing for myself – playing music, cooking, petting our cats, reading, watching beautiful sunrises and sunsets, feeling the soft new spring growth on the pine tree in our back yard, contemplating the voluptuousness of the many irises that grace our gardens, and listening to the sound of the small waterfall in our pond outside our porch. I could go on and on. Just starting this list is a reminder that I do many, many things for myself. The trick is to pay attention to them. So the next time my friend asks, "What are you doing for yourself?" I will pause, take a deep breath and say, "I'm paying attention." Then I will rattle off some of the things that have touched my heart because I have, indeed, been paying attention.

Despite everything Bennett has gone through, he seems much better at living a balanced life than I do. In his CarePages you can glimpse how much he enjoys and loves life. If I'm not careful, I succumb to wallowing in worry. Bennett, on the other hand, sees worry as a waste of imagination (he learned that from a fellow cancer survivor), and he continues to relish life – the best way to survive cancer day by day.

Reflection #3 (fall/winter 2011)

Little Things

Paying attention to life means more than taking time to absorb and appreciate the wonderful, big things that happen. Those are easy to take in and cherish. Equally as important is paying attention to little things – the small miracles that greet us every day if we take the time to stop and widen the circle of our attention.

The little things that arrest my attention are the ones that play with my senses. The velvety softness of new leaves in the spring, the sparkle of a thousand tiny prisms on the dew-covered morning lawn, the aroma of Bennett's spaghetti sauce followed by the mixture of spices and textures on my tongue, the chirping of a bright red cardinal perched on a snowy white branch, the sublime turn of a phrase in Mozart's string quintets – the world engages me in hundreds of sensual experiences every day. My obligation in this contract we call life is to notice them and let them fill me with awe.

Little things and small moments are easy to miss. I've found that paying attention to them makes every day with cancer easier to survive.

I Don't Know How to Do This

Sometimes the feeling of "I don't know how to do this" washes over me, and no amount of breathing deeply, letting go of worry, and paying attention to little things helps. I feel pulled under by the horrible weight of the unknown and, at the same time, I feel guilty for not being stronger. Swallowing my fears because I don't want my negative energy depleting Bennett's determination makes me feel even worse. Sometimes drinking a glass or two of red wine seems to offer some temporary relief. And sleeping can take away the pain, but it's back again when I wake up.

I felt the same "I don't know how to do this" when my mother was dying. I could find no map that would help me navigate the terrifying terrain of losing someone I loved so much. From that experience I learned that to go through this current uncertain and difficult time, I need to accept the rush of conflicting feelings, accept the tears, and accept that "I don't know how to do this." Knowing how to do it or not, I am being forced to do it.

I am reminded of the words of the Spanish poet Antonio Machado:

O traveler, there is no path
Paths are made by walking.

As Bennett and I walk this path of surviving cancer today and then walk it again tomorrow, I find that that path we are making is much like a spiral or a labyrinth. It's not a straight line; it doesn't get easier as we keep going. The path circles around itself, and I relive experiences and feelings that I thought I had left behind. At other times something new – a new perspective, a new challenge, a new insight – appears just around the corner. Through it all I keep walking, learning "how to do this" as I go.

Faith

When my husband and I were cleaning out my Mom's apartment after she died, we discovered a number of small inspirational pamphlets that she had collected over the years. I knew she had frequently found strength in reading the daily devotional guide *The Upper Room*, but I wasn't aware she had filled her desk and bureau drawers with tiny books of quotations from the Bible and accompanying commentary to help her get through the years of my dad's declining health and death. I saved some of them, and now I find myself turning to the same verses. The words are a source of great hope and strength.

The verse that meant the most to her and now sustains me as well is Isaiah 40:31: "But they who wait for the Lord shall renew their strength, they shall mount up with wings like eagles, they shall run and not be weary, they shall walk and not faint." I remember her telling me that it was this verse that kept her going. These days it does the same for me.

I long to have my mother here to help me through this journey of surviving cancer with Bennett. We used to talk at least once a day, and although it's been almost ten years since she died, I miss her every day. But I feel her presence, not just in the Bible verses we share, but also in the many reminders of the bond of love that still exists between us. The sweet-smelling lilac bush blooming outside the patio door in the room where she slept when she stayed with us, messages on little gift cards she sent me when she was alive that I discover in unexpected places, the hawk that passes overhead when I'm thinking about her – all of these and more let me know she is here. More than anything else it is in the everyday miracles of nature that I feel her presence most strongly. It is those same miracles that ground my faith in the One who loves us.

My husband and I offer prayers of gratitude every evening. We also ask for healing and strength for us and others. Knowing that our prayers for Bennett are echoed by many, we give thanks for being surrounded by loving family and friends. Responses to Bennett's CarePages are filled with prayers for his continued strength and well-being along with requests for divine guidance for doctors' wisdom.

Many times throughout the day I find myself turning to God and praying for comfort and support. Giving voice to my desperation and feeling listened to, I know I am not traveling this journey alone. I know that under God's wings, I "will find refuge" (Psalm 91:4).

Embrace Life with Gratitude

There are times – moments that sometimes stretch into days – when worry takes over, robbing me of the precious time that Bennett and I have together. What I have resolved to do instead of worrying is to embrace every moment of my life with gratitude. It's more than paying attention; it's accompanying my act of attention with a deep thankfulness for all that I encounter along the way. When I fill up my moments with gratitude, there is no room left for worry.

This practice of offering thanks is more than uttering a quick "thank you" for the blessings that surround me. It is pausing to peel back the layers of the existence in which I am embedded at any particular moment. For example, right now I'm sitting at the computer typing these words. When I pause to consider what I have to be grateful for in the present moment, my list is endless. It's important to name some of them – the warm room in which I sit, the window by my desk that offers me a tree-house view of trees and low mountains, the home that we are lucky enough to own, my husband who works at his desk right behind me, my two cats who are now sleeping in a nearby chair but who sometimes nudge me away from my typing, and the electricity that I'm using to power my computer and the light that shines on my pages. How fortunate I am to live in this beautiful place!

Then there are my fingers that are able to hit the keys fairly accurately and are still able to pull music from a violin. There's my mind that helps me form these words, my eyes that help me see them, my ears that help me arrange them, and my heart that helps me envision others. How lucky I am to have this body with which to create and experience! Then there are all the people who have held me and guided me – a father who gave up every one of his Saturday afternoons and Monday evenings to take me to music lessons and rehearsals, a mother who loved me no matter what, and grandmothers who taught me to love music and the earth. How immensely blessed I am to have had parents and grandparents who loved and cared for me. Then there are the people who labor to make the clothes and objects in my life and others who work to grow and transport the food I eat. How often I take them for granted! How privileged I am!

At this point, I pause to match my gratitude with resolve for action on behalf of peace and justice. My recognition of the endless things for which I am called to express thanks reminds me of what I need to give back in return.

A few days ago I made a commitment to myself to transform every worry into a call for gratitude. I can't say that I have alchemized worry into thankfulness 100% of the time, but my practice of giving thanks has filled my life with a profound realization of the blessings that uphold my life. Each moment I spend in embracing life with gratitude fills me with love, and that love is so much more important to give to Bennett than my worry.

Reflection #4 (fall/winter 2011)

*L*ightly

During a particularly difficult time in our marriage, Bennett and I worked separately with two wonderful and wise counselors. Both were brilliant and helped us beyond what we, or they, could imagine at the time. In one of my sessions in which I was describing the weight I felt on my shoulders from trying to live up to my belief that others expected me to be perfect, my counselor suggested that I wear that expectation more "lightly" – replace the weight of expectation, worry, fear, anger, etc. with a gossamer shawl that barely touched my shoulders. What a relief! The situation that brought up my reaction was still there, but "wearing it lightly" cast it in a new light, and I could deal with it without becoming weighed down and entangled in drama.

I've used his prescription to "wear it lightly" when confronted with bad news about Bennett's cancer. It doesn't diminish the seriousness of the diagnosis, but it does help me to hear it and live with it from a far less frantic and fearful place. I remembered this remark when Bennett was experiencing the devastating side effects of chemotherapy, not to make light of them, but to lighten my load so that I could be more helpful to Bennett. When I wear this journey of surviving cancer "lightly," I can face all that happens along the way without wearing down this traveler. And when I do that, my husband gains a traveling companion who is wholly and fully present.

*I*mages

We wouldn't have known Bennett had lung cancer if it hadn't of been for a chance CT scan taken when he was in the hospital for what the doctors thought might be a heart problem. It revealed a very small tumor in his right lung. That scan and the PET scan that followed did not reveal that the cancer was also in a lymph node. The surgeon found that during surgery. Scans – images – are not perfect.

CT and PET scans have now indicated that there is a recurrence of Bennett's lung cancer in three small lymph nodes in his chest. Actually, the images indicated something suspicious; the biopsy determined they were malignant. Images do not tell all, but we are glad that they tell something. Unfortunately, they do not tell us what to do. We can only make our best guess about treatment options, and then go forward without looking back.

For the past several Christmases, my husband and I have sent out e-card holiday messages with a snippet of a recording from one of our recent concerts and a photograph of the two of us taken after the performance. Friends tell us that they like the music, and this year, they remarked that we both look so happy. But images can reveal and hide at the same time. We are happy. We're happy that we have the opportunity to perform and play together. We're happy that the audience appeared to enjoy the performance. And when it comes right down to it, we're basically happy people. What the photo does not reveal is everything we pushed below the surface in order to pull off the performance. It doesn't show the worry and the fear nor does it capture the anger and the frustration regarding the cancer returning. Images hide what we ourselves do not want to reveal. Or do they?

As I look at photographs of myself as well as photos of family and friends, I am struck by what they can capture – how the slightest hint of a frown and the miniscule bending of a shoulder seem to reveal persistent body pain, how the tilt of the head coupled with a somewhat restrained smile in a graduation picture seem to indicate wistfulness about what the future may bring, and how a firm stance and upward thrust of the head seem to suggest a strong determination in the face of life's challenges. But perhaps I'm reading too much into the images.

When the oncologist showed us images from Bennett's diagnostic scans, both my husband and I wondered at how anyone could read them. Maybe it is just like reading a photograph of dear friends. We do it with our minds and our hearts. Perhaps for doctors, it's the same. We want them to draw on all of their experience, wisdom and intuition, see below the surface of the image, and issue a definitive reading – the cancer is here and no other place. And if they target and destroy the cancer they do see with radiation, we can be sure that the cancer exists no where else in my husband's body. Right? Wrong!

I believe that scans, like photographs, are not reality. They are an image of reality. We can gather knowledge from them – knowledge that is sifted through our own experiences and relationships with the people in the photos and knowledge that is informed by everything we bring to the diagnostic process. But in the end, they don't tell us everything. The story of the picture emerges from a mysterious collaboration between image and viewer. Looking at the happy couple in our e-card, I imagine their story. Looking at my husband's scans, the doctors imagine his. Who is to say what is really there.

Fight

Bennett has a lot of fight in him. He can be as tenacious as a bull dog. Cancer couldn't have a more determined, hard-hitting adversary.

I've seen Bennett fight on a lot of occasions. In fact I think it was this ability of his to stand up to opponents, think quickly on his feet, and out maneuver them with on-the-spot, well-thought out arguments that first attracted me to him. As I watched him devour his colleagues in faculty meetings, I couldn't help but be impressed with this man who could land verbal knockout punches so quickly and with such ease. I know that he's doing the same with cancer.

*E*nergy

It takes energy to perform. Not frenetic, run-around-the-room, multitasking energy, but focused, concentrated, life-carrying energy. It's energy born of the intention to create something new and the commitment to sustain it. It's life-giving and life-affirming, and it's also a deep mystery.

I was sitting next to my mother when she took her last breath. One moment she was there; the next she wasn't. Somewhere between the inhale and exhale, the life energy that was her left her body. I was overwhelmed with the feeling that she hadn't just disappeared. There was no way that her strong life force had simply evaporated into thin air. I knew that her energy, in some form that remains a mystery to me, continued to exist and continues to exist to this day.

I am also aware of life's energy when I practice tai chi, have acupuncture, meditate and pray. When a friend tells me about the joys and sorrows in her life, I can feel her energy change. My husband and I read each other's energy without thought. At times, we read each other better than we read ourselves. Sometimes in nature – working in the garden or walking through the woods – I feel as if life is all energy. In those moments, there is no separation between me and everything that I take in with my senses. Everything is seamlessly connected. Remembering such intimacy during difficult times, I summon courage and strength by drawing energy from the earth.

At various times in his cancer journey, Bennett has worked with healers who move energy. He has experienced pain relief as well as emotional comfort in these sessions. Their efforts may have helped keep the cancer at bay for the past two years. Hopefully their work will continue to give him strength to continue to survive cancer day after day. Friends and family repeatedly tell Bennett that they are sending him healing energy. And we know that these gifts have kept his spirits up and his body going.

There is an energy that enlivens our bodies. The same energy lights up every intimate exchange with the world that surrounds and nurtures us. It connects the hearts of family and friends who carry a deep love for one another, and it supports our bodies' tremendous power to heal itself. The source of this energy is the greatest mystery of all.

Reflection #5 (fall/winter 2011)

Listening

I find playing string quartets to be one of life's greatest pleasures. At its best, the experience is transcendent, and I lose myself in the musical conversation. Intimately attuned to one another and the music, we create a single organism as each of us takes turns leading then following, suggesting a new musical nuance then taking one up, fitting into or dominating the musical texture, and shaping the drama of the music without uttering a word. How does this happen? It is accomplished by listening so acutely that we feel we are one. Frankly, and I'm far from the first person to say this, playing chamber music can be as good as, and sometimes better than, sex. In both I listen and am listened to in such a way that everything drops away except the lovemaking – the music – itself.

Surviving cancer day by day requires listening at this same deep level. Listening to his body helped Bennett discern what treatment to follow, what food to eat and what advice to heed. When his body told him he had had enough chemo, he listened to it. Listening to my husband hash out his feelings and fears, I have been included as a survivor in this cancer journey. Listening to me has helped Bennett not worry quite so much about me, which leaves him free to focus on his own healing needs. Listening to the members of his cancer support group and being listened to by others who are traveling the same cancer journey has helped Bennett face many of the challenges he has encountered along the way. When my friends listen to me, just listen, I feel honored in the place where I am, not in the place they think I should be.

Listening closely is an art. It requires the listener suspend judgment, resist the temptation to tell one's own story, and simply get out of the way. Listening is extremely difficult to do. In the chamber group of professionals and amateurs that I direct, listening to each other is sometimes elusive. One has to have such a mastery of the music and oneself that it is possible to let both go and lose oneself in the interplay of sound and musical line. It is the same in a spoken conversation. If I'm listening just to me, how can I enter even the shallowest level of intimacy with a friend? Neither the music, nor the friendship, will flourish.

This kind of listening as an act of honoring the speaker is essential in a doctor-patient relationship. Bennett has been blessed with a surgeon and an oncologist who really listen to him. Not only do they take the time to listen to what he is saying and respond thoughtfully to what he is asking, they have taken the time to get to know my husband in a way that informs their listening. Upon these thoughtful exchanges a mountain of trust has been built, and I know that this trust has helped my husband survive cancer.

Listening opens hearts to each other and to life. As we have listened to the love in friends' hearts and as they have lovingly listened to our pain and our fear, we have heard their concern and felt their compassion. It is this kind of listening that has filled our surviving with immeasurable joy.

Intuition

Knowing how to navigate this journey of surviving cancer with Bennett has often been a matter of intuition – listening to my inner knowing and trusting what I hear. It can be easy to discount this internal direction. Sometimes it is so subtle, so imperceptible, I wonder if it is imagined. Yet every time I ignore it, I discover its authenticity.

Knowing without thought usually comes to me unbidden. Although I don't seem to be able to summon such knowing, I have learned to pay attention to intuition when it nudges me at the edges of my consciousness. When that happens, I know that this is what I need to heed. This is what I need to notice. This is what I need to say. This is when I need to be silent. And most importantly, this is how I can best help my husband.

My desire for omnipotence seems to hold intuition's visits at bay. I want to make the cancer go away. I wish it had never made an appearance. I want the needle to go painlessly into my husband's arm. I want the nausea to disappear. I wish I could give him strength. I want to make it easier on him. I don't want to worry Bennett with my worry. I wish I was stronger so he wouldn't see my fear. I wish I knew just what to do. Why can't I do all this and more?

Taking a deep breath, I accept that I can't. What I can do is listen to that knowing voice within and do what I can. Tonight we're going to set up a massage table that we borrowed from a friend, and I'm going to give Bennett Reiki in hopes of minimizing the effects of the radiation and chemotherapy treatments that he just started. He asked how often we should do these sessions. I told him his intuition will help him know when and how often. We are both learning to trust the knowing that lives beyond words.

Friends

I find the number of friends on Bennett's CarePages astonishing – 102! And this doesn't count the 98 friends to whom he sends separate email updates. This support network includes people we see regularly where we live and friends that Bennett has collected along the way throughout his life. Among the most amazing are his former students. Many of them have let him know that he has made an enormous difference in their lives. Their moving comments on CarePages and in individual emails are truly heart-warming. Bennett is uplifted by all of them, and they have truly carried both of us along on his surviving cancer journey.

Bennett has been exceedingly grateful for the deepening of friendships as well as the renewal of old friendships. There are several of these close friends who call often to see how he's doing and to offer their support and encouragement. Friends in town come to sit with him during the worst chemo days, and we have a refrigerator overflowing with chicken soup! Being surrounded by this extended family has helped Bennett get through many tough times over the past several years.

They have also helped me – by listening, by giving me a break from care giving, by cooking, by sending me funny emails, and by giving me good, strong hugs. Both Bennett and I feel blessed by the love of so many. If there is a silver lining in this difficult journey, we have found one in the deepening bonds of friendship to the friends we knew we had and the rekindled connections to the friends we thought had disappeared forever from our lives. We are lucky to have each and every one of them.

*E*scape

Sometimes no amount of listening with understanding, cooking healthy food, sending me uplifting notes, or hugging me tightly around my shoulders is what I feel I need. Sometimes I just need to escape from everyone and everything. I have three main escape routes – nature, books and wine. The first two are probably much better for me than the last one.

I have always found solace in nature. Since I was a child I have been enchanted by flowers and stones, trees and mountains, shells and waves breaking on the shore. There is a wonderful photograph of me as a two-year old bending over a bed of flowers. In it, I appear to be talking to a flower that is touching my nose. Now sixty years later, I still find myself talking to flowers as well as everything else in the natural world. I think the only way I made it through the grueling years of doctoral study was the pine tree I befriended in the university parking lot on my way to spending endless hours in the library. And the irises in my garden continue to comfort me as they remind me of my mother's presence.

On many days during this cancer journey, I find that the simple act of looking out my study window onto grass and trees and hills and sky connects me with the earth. When I was young, I spent a small portion of many summers on my grandparents' farm in western Montana, and I think that these weeks spent in a beautiful valley in the Rockies infused my being with a longing for space that only the generous vistas of wide valleys and towering mountains can fulfill. From both grandmothers I learned to live in close dialogue with dirt and the beings embedded in it. Enmeshed in the natural world, I can breathe long enough to find respite from the troubles of this journey with cancer.

I also escape into books. I've been an avid reader all of my life. Growing up an only child, I found friends and refuge in the worlds that I visited through words. When the real world that surrounded me was uncertain, I found particular relief in mysteries. So it is again. Prior to this current round of chemo and radiation, I set out on a project to read a biography of every American president. As fascinating as these stories are, I can't seem to lose myself in them the same way I can forget myself in the prose of a beautifully written mystery – a good mystery, not a gory one. I lose myself so completely that I find I have to ration my reading or else I can spend whole days doing nothing but reading. As one friend reminds me, there could be worse ways of escaping.

Another friend says the same thing about drinking wine. I've grown really fond of Spanish reds and, at the end of hard days, I look forward to a glass or two. Honestly, I look forward to how a glass or two helps me escape the bad scenes the day might have held and the worry that grew up around them. A couple of glasses don't make them go away, but they do help me escape into a state of non-worry.

As I write this, I am struck that my need to escape is selfish. I cannot even begin to imagine how it is to have cancer and want to escape. What I do know is that I struggle, sometimes more mightily than others, to remain present to my husband, his needs and the demands of this journey. But there are times after taking care of him in which I imagine nothing better than putting myself in some other place where I don't have to think about the cancer or do anything about it. I can't help but think that upon returning from such escapes, I am better able to face what needs to be done in order for both of us to continue on this journey.

Reflection #6 (winter 2011-2012)

*L*ight

When we lived in Miami, Bennett loved the warm weather because he could play golf year-round. I missed the seasons. During our first year in Florida, there were moments when I actually had to stop and ask myself whether it was fall, winter or spring. The sunlight didn't seem to change very much. Gradually, however, I learned that if I paid more attention to the quality of the sunlight, I could discover remarkable seasonal changes. I found that the light in the winter is astonishingly soft, and I grew to love tracking its subtle contrasts. It's really only in late spring that the sunlight assumes the sheering, white intensity of the light I once thought "normal" for south Florida. There are seasons. I just had to learn to be more observant.

When we moved from Florida to Maryland and then to West Virginia, I had my seasons back, but I lost some of the special feeling I got when Miami's winter sun made the world a little softer. Here in Berkeley Springs the sun's oblique rays cast much longer shadows in the winter, and there is a grayness that seems to envelop the world from solstice to equinox. During these months, my body thirsts for more light. When we visit friends and family in Florida in January or February, I can't get enough of the sun. In contrast to what I've left in West Virginia, it shines yellow and bright. I thought of shades of sunlight the other day when I looked at Bennett's face the evening of his first day of chemo and fourth day of radiation. The light in his face had changed. He was paler than usual. He felt OK and was coping reasonably well with the nausea and tiredness, but I could tell from the color of his complexion that his body had experienced the trauma of chemotherapy. How remarkable it is that we can discern such subtle differences in those we love! I know that I can detect minute changes in Bennett's body language, speaking tone, walking tempo, skin texture, and eye color. I just wish I could sense the disappearance of cancer in his body. And I really wish that I could make the cancer disappear completely.

Remembering the feeling of the south Florida sun on my light-starved face, I know that light and energy have healing powers. So although I can't reach in and take out the cancer, I can envision the bright sunlight filling my husband's chest with all the creative, life-enhancing energy that the Creator can muster. That is something I can do, and when many of our friends tell Bennett that they are sending him light and love, I know they are doing the same.

Identity

My father struggled with many health problems in the final decade of his life. During one of these challenging times when he was recovering in the assisted-living section of the retirement community where he and my mother were living, he became the Dad I wished I could have had around more often when I was growing up. For a few weeks he became a gentle and caring man, not the angry and sometimes bitter man that my mom and I were used to seeing. I don't know if it was the drugs, the situation, a sudden chemical change, or something else. All I know was that for the first time in my life, I could sit with my father and have a conversation. Even his facial expression and the look in his eyes had changed. There was no evidence of the fear and rage that usually rested just below the surface. I treasured and continue to treasure those few weeks with my father, for all too soon and without warning or any identifiable cause, he was back to the short-tempered man I had known most of my life.

I think some of my Dad's personality changes must have been the result of medications he was taking. I've also seen personality changes in Bennett. Two years ago when he was recovering from two surgeries and trying to make it through chemotherapy, the pain killers and the anti-nausea drugs he was taking wrecked havoc on his body and mind. My husband is an emotionally strong, stalwart, and determinedly optimistic man. The medications not only weakened his already weak body, they reduced him to a trembling, tearful man who was afraid of everything. Bennett became non-Bennett. I think it was this identity change along with his incredibly diminished quality of life that convinced Bennett to halt further chemotherapy. Once the chemicals left his body – it took more than several months – Bennett gradually recovered his strength and his feisty nature.

Now two years later as he begins a new course of chemotherapy, we are taking the oncologist at his word. The doctor has promised that he will try his best not to have chemo reduce Bennett to, in his words, "a puddle." We will have to see what the next seven weeks bring. In the meantime, Bennett is Bennett for most of the time. Morning nausea still chips around the edges of his resolute personality, but by lunchtime he's back to being the man who is determined to practice the trumpet and walk two miles every day.

Forgiveness

I wish I had forgiven my father when he was alive. Letting go of my internal anger at his external anger would have made me a much more compassionate daughter during the final difficult years of his life. Over the decade since his death, I've learned how to balance the good of our relationship with those awful times when my mom and I were reduced to tears because of his anger. The fulcrum of that balancing act is forgiveness. It doesn't make the bad stuff disappear nor does it excuse it. Forgiveness keeps the memory of what was bad in our relationship from outweighing the good.

Bennett and I have forgiven each other much during our more than three decades together. We've had to. We're human. Without forgiveness our love wouldn't have survived.

Part of my journey of surviving cancer is forgiving Bennett for not giving up smoking years before he eventually stopped. I pestered him to stop, and he would give it up from time to time, but he would always start up again. I have a clear memory of saying to him that if he ever ended up with lung cancer, I would be incredibly angry and would never speak to him again. My threats didn't do any good. It took a couple of bouts with pneumonia to convince him to throw away his cigarettes permanently. And it took my declaration to never kiss him again if he didn't give up cigars to persuade him to surrender all of his smoking addictions. He still laughs when he tells the story of how I timed my ultimatum – he had just walked into our house with several bundles of premium cigars he had purchased on a business trip to New Orleans. Keeping my fingers crossed that Bennett loved kissing me more than he liked smoking great cigars, I told him it was either me or the cigars. He made the right choice. The next day he packed up all of his cigars and cigar paraphernalia and mailed them to friends.

I've reneged on my threat about never speaking to him now that he has lung cancer. Of course my threat was juvenile and silly, but I do remember the depth of my anger at Bennett for not chucking the cigarettes when I asked him to stop. I forgave him then because on balance, there was more good in our young relationship than bad. Now thirty years later, we've tipped the scales so heavily on the good side that forgiveness comes very quickly.

*E*ffort

I was floored by the amount of effort it took me to make it through just one day during the months Bennett was dealing with the aftermath of lung surgery, the emergency need for a second surgery, the side effects of chemo, and the side effects from the drugs meant to counteract the chemo side effects. The effort to care for him as well as watch after the house, the garden, meals, laundry, bills, and our consulting business was overwhelming. I was extremely lucky that I didn't have to take care of children as well. I don't know how mothers with children manage when their husbands are surviving cancer. It must be exponentially more difficult.

For me the difficulty arose because "normally" we divide our home and business tasks equally, but with Bennett's incapacitation, all those tasks fell squarely on my shoulder. The more I tried to keep up with them, the more flustered and frustrated I became. I had to let some of them slide, knowing that I would eventually work through all of them with the help of family and friends. I also believed that eventually Bennett would regain his strength, and we would divvy up the chores once again.

Applying more effort to a difficult situation doesn't always make it better. Trying harder to ignore the water that I have to cross to get to the green usually ends in a bad golf swing and my ball in the water. Trying harder to find the rhythmic groove as I apply my classical violin technique to Celtic fiddling usually results in a lurching dance tune. In many situations I've found that it's better if I trust my body to execute my desired intentions. Most of the time this works, particularly when I remain unattached to the results. Therein lies the difficulty – how to remain unattached when I want the results to be good. Wanting to play the fiddle well is one thing. Wanting my husband to survive cancer is quite another. How do I remain unattached to that result?

I can't. But I can learn to apply my effort to what needs doing right now – making dinner for example – reminding myself that my husband is alive right now. At the same time, I can get my mind, my worry, out of the way and let my body do what it knows how to do. If I lose myself in the task at hand, it takes much less effort. If I lose myself in a series of tasks – all those things I need to get done – then, one by one, they get done and surviving cancer takes a little less effort.

Reflection #7 (winter 2011-2012)

*L*aughter

Laughter. What could be better! Silly email jokes that friends send us, uproariously funny comedy routines on TV, news that we just cannot believe, and our cats' antics that my cousin astutely describes as "a circus of joy" can tickle a few gentle chuckles or side-splitting, hearty guffaws. What a delight it is to be swallowed up by laughter and then spit out into a new world a little bit fresher and a tiny bit renewed.

Much has been written about the benefits of laughter. For us, laughter is a release and a reminder – a release from the worry that can sometime overtake us and a reminder that we can still feel good in the midst of these challenging times. It feels really good to feel good.

Experiencing something funny together also connects us to each other in the present as well as the past. It brings to our bodies, if perhaps not to our minds, memories of all the other times we've shared good laughs and good times. Laughing out loud with my husband, I am transported to a place where "all is right with the world." And during those moments of laughing together, it is.

I Do

After Bennett's first surgery when the surgeon told me that my husband's cancer was stage III and not stage I, I wasn't sure he'd be alive in two years for our 30th anniversary. As I listened to the grim statistics associated with the reclassification, I prayed that Bennett would make it to January 2012. Thankfully he did, and this week we're celebrating our 30th. While his cancer has recurred, Bennett has managed the radiation and chemotherapy treatments so unbelievably well that we have been able to have a wonderful celebratory lunch at one of our favorite restaurants. I realize now that I asked for far too little time so I've amended my prayers and am asking God to help us both greet our 50th anniversary with healthy bodies and minds!

Bennett has never troubled himself with survival rate statistics, and I've come to adopt his "they don't apply to me" attitude. Both his surgeon and his oncologist have made it a point to assure us that Bennett is an individual and that numbers cannot predict how his cancer will play out. Both doctors have stayed away from discussing numbers with us because they say that they don't want them to "play with our heads." In the early days of our cancer journey, I failed to follow their lead, and I let the statistics regarding five-year survival rates that I discovered on the Internet play around with my head far more than was good for me. I have had to learn that as far as Bennett's future is concerned, they are meaningless. He means to confound the statistics and break all records. That he's surviving with the same dogged determination and hopeful optimism that he brought to keeping our marriage together for thirty years in spite of some pretty tough times is a testament to his life view that sees everything as possible.

*F*inished

Bennett just finished the last of his thirty-five radiation treatments, and the seven chemotherapy sessions ended a week ago. The nurses gave him a certificate that indicated that he graduated with "high honors," and he brought them donuts to celebrate (not the healthiest of treats, but definitely fun).

His experience undergoing both treatments at the same time has been much better than what we anticipated given the dire warnings from the radiation oncologist of possible side effects. Only in the last few days has the cumulative effects of the radiation made it extremely difficult for him to swallow. Thankfully that condition has been helped with a couple of hours of intravenous fluids and some pretty powerful painkillers. Bennett's hoping that he won't have to take the medications for too long, but for now, they're helping him swallow enough liquids to keep his body hydrated.

Along with the nurses and the doctors, Bennett attributes his body's ability to cope with the tough 7-week regimen to exercising (he walked 2+ miles on a treadmill every day), drinking a lot of water (3+ liters), and remaining positive and optimistic throughout the entire episode except for two days when dehydration reduced him to a "puddle." Today when I took him for his last treatment, his nurse, the technician and several patients that we have gotten to know because they share the same treatment time commented to me that Bennett exudes strength, good humor and optimism. We are all convinced that it is these qualities that have kept him going.

Speaking of other patients, I have been inspired by the courage and determination I have witnessed in so many people who have shared the chemo room and waiting spaces with us. Their kindness and caring wishes have certainly helped to carry us through these challenging weeks.

The nurses and technicians have been simply fantastic. Their skill at sticking Bennett relatively painlessly, their patience in answering our questions, their concern for his comfort and well-being, their advice on how to counteract side effects, and their compassionate words of support have been immeasurably helpful. We could not be making this journey without them. They have our deepest gratitude.

In a month and a half, Bennett will have a CT scan to look at the troublesome lymph nodes that were the target of this round of chemo and radiation. I refuse to use the "C" word when talking about them, because by now I know that they are harmless! Both of us choose to spend our moments in the land of no "C." One could call it denial. We call it reveling in the life that we have together right now. We toasted that commitment yesterday on Valentine's Day (a glass of red wine for me and water for Bennett). We gave an even bigger "hurrah" for the end of radiation/chemo and the beginning of what comes next.

*E*mergency

Sometimes surviving cancer feels like I'm waiting for the other shoe to drop. Is his cough from pneumonia? Is his sudden weakness from an infection? When Bennett has some sort of a health problem – a prolonged sneezing attack, unexplained aches and pains, a more severe than usual attack of reflux – my first thought is that the cancer has returned with a vengeance. That is what I thought the other day when it really did feel like the other shoe had dropped. We were in the "Express Admissions Unit" of the hospital waiting for a room to become available. I had taken Bennett to the hospital because he was suffering from uncontrollable chills, shaking and shortness of breath.

We're now four days down the road since I wrote the last paragraph, and Bennett is still in the hospital. He's feeling better though, and it looks like he'll be going home tomorrow. For a time, the other shoe did fall. We're still not entirely out of the woods – they haven't identified the cause of his symptoms and his descending white blood cell count (it started to go in the good direction just this morning) – but he's feeling much better, and we know that he will continue to improve much more quickly at home than in the hospital.

Bennett and I have been theorizing about why the other shoe fell this past week. He sailed through chemotherapy and seven weeks of radiation. Why would the shoe fall now after two weeks? We think that his body was just worn out from fighting – first the therapies and then the pain medications for the esophageal burn. It was just too much, and even his determination and positive attitude were worn out. Thankfully after four days in the hospital, his body is starting to rebound.

How does it feel when the shoe is dropping? How do I feel when I don't know why he's feeling so miserable, why his white blood cell count is declining or what can be done about it or what's going to happen? It feels as if I have become unmoored. I'm consumed with fear over what is happening and what the future might bring. It also feels as if my self is divided – the scared one who wants someone to take charge and make it all right again, and the strong one who knows that I might be able to help my husband turn the corner towards recovery if I model strength and confidence. It's the strong one who went into his hospital room on day three and gently, yet firmly, got him up and moving around, and convinced him that he would feel better if he shaved and cleaned up a little. As a good friend suggested, if we can get his body doing some normal activities, maybe we can trick it into returning to some semblance of normalcy. What helps when the shoe is dropping? Once again it's friends and family. They brought love and support for both of us into Bennett's hospital room. They also brought nutritious food, a collection of vitamins and nutrients for strength and ginger for nausea. We know that their presence, calls, emails and prayers have helped lift the shoe up again.

Good news also helps to lift the shoe. In looking for the cause of this episode, the doctor ordered a new CT scan, which revealed that the lymph nodes have shrunk. Hallelujah! All of Bennett's body's hard work, all of the love and prayers that have been sent his way, all of the good food that he has eaten, all of Bennett's towering will to heal, and yes, all of that poisonous chemo and radiation have done what we hoped they would do. All along we've said that we didn't care what worked. We just wanted something to work. This is good news, indeed!

Will I go back to feeling as if I'm waiting for the other shoe to drop? Probably. But I'll try to remember what I've written in other places in these reflections – be thankful for this blessed moment – this moment when I'm sitting next to my husband whose body is coming back to health.

Reflection #8 (summer 2012)

*L*istening

Listening takes as much practice as making music. In fact, listening is an integral part of making music, and you can't make music – and you can't live life – if you don't listen. It's one of the things that has helped us survive cancer.

Bennett listening to his body. Both of us listening to each other – really listening by putting aside our preoccupations and our preconceived notions of what the other person might need and giving each other the space to say what's on our minds. Listening to our intuition regarding what food to eat and what natural remedies might help. Listening to the advice of others and filtering out what is not helpful. Listening to our gut feelings about what might be causing the pain that has plagued Bennett for five months – pain that a barrage of medical tests have been unable to explain. Listening to the subtle changes of tone and inflection in Bennett's voice to give me clues about how he's feeling. Listening to how our automatic reactions to stress and uncertainty sometimes spill over into words and actions we wish we had kept to ourselves. Listening to the daily messages of love we send to each other that tend to get overlooked in the busyness of preparing meals, doing chores and surviving cancer. All of this listening requires paying attention and letting go of the chatter that frequently surrounds our lives.

Listening unties the knot of fear that rests somewhere under my ribs. It doesn't diminish the possibility of cancer's return, but it does make the present moment a treasure beyond compare.

In Sickness and in Health

There is no way to be prepared for the "in sickness" part of marriage. No way to come to a new "normal," as some have recommend. The only way through it for me is to let go the notion of any kind of "normal."

But I like "normal." I like "happily every after." I like everything settled and in its place. I liked our life before cancer. How can I come to like our new life surviving cancer?

The answer lies in the word "like." It's the wrong word. The marriage vows that Bennett and I took 30 years ago didn't say "to like from this day forward." They said "to have and to hold from this day forward." "Having" and "holding" are essential because marriage, and life, are not going to be filled with only good times – times that are easy to "like." Our marriage has included the good and the bad – "for better or for worse, for richer, for poorer, in sickness and in health." Bennett and I have learned that we must "have" and "hold" each other no matter what circumstances come our way.

Having been married once before, I readily admit that sometimes there's not enough love left to "have and to hold" – to stick with each other through thick and thin. Sometimes the well of love that once sustained a marriage runs dry, and there are no springs to replenish it. In this long marriage that Bennett and I have shared, there have been times when the well has gotten pretty low, so low that for a while I wasn't sure whether or not I wanted the well to fill up again. On the other hand, Bennett has always been sure. For my part, what fills the well up again is our history of "having" and "holding" through good times and bad. It is a deep and holy appreciation for our shared life together that helps the springs of love start to bubble up again.

In our surviving cancer journey there is no shortage of water in the well; there's just the recognition that our life together has been irrevocably changed. What we do together has changed. Some things we'll never do again. How we do things has changed. The context in which we live has changed. But Bennett and I still "have" and "hold" each other – we attend to each other with the fullest devotion that we can muster. If there are days when Bennett, because of pain, can only muster a small amount, I figure I can "have" and "hold" tight enough for both of us.

Fidelity

Fidelity is an old-fashioned word. In this era of fast everything – food, travel, communication, and gratification – the idea of steadfastness, constancy and attachment seems anachronistic. The notion of fidelity seems much too slow – much too stuck – for the world in which we live. But "stickiness" is exactly what it takes for us to survive cancer day by day. The "adherence to something to which one is bound by a pledge or duty" is precisely how we make it through every moment of every day. Our allegiance to each other, the stickiness and messiness of our long-lived love for each other, is the glue that keeps us together. The measure of our devotion is our absolute unwillingness to let cancer dissolve that glue – no matter how many tears, no matter how hard the struggle, no matter how strong the desire for a life without uncertainty.

Recently I've been going through a box of my mother's things – letters, photographs, her family Bible, her diaries from high school, her father's diaries (they're in Swedish, and I'm sad that I can't read them), cards from me that she saved, and some of her jewelry. She died nine years ago, and it's only now that I am able to savor these reminders of her without needing a box of Kleenex by my side. I find comfort in knowing that the "stickiness" of my relationship with my Mom helps to fill the hole in my heart caused by her passing.

But it wasn't my mother that drew me to the box. It was the typewritten story of my great-grandmother and her life in Sweden, the voyage to America with her husband, children and other close family, and their pioneering life in Minnesota as told by my grandmother's sister that called me to the box's contents. Her tale of dreams and hardships overcome testify to the courage it takes to remain steadfast in the midst of the most trying, difficult and heart-breaking conditions. I found the same tenacity in my grandmother's letters. Surely it was fidelity and faith that made it possible for my grandmother to keep going when, within the space of two days, she lost her 8-year old daughter and 5-year old son to flu while 8-months pregnant with my mom's older sister. And she did this without my grandfather for he had gone to Montana to look for land to homestead.

Today as I walk this journey of surviving cancer with Bennett, I wish I could sit down with my grandmother and ask her how she did it. I'd like to ask my father's mother the same question. She endured her own share of loss and a husband's extended illness while having to do most of the work to maintain their farm in western Montana. Both of my grandmothers had to make it through the Depression with little or no money. How did they do it? How did they keep on keeping on?

I know for certain that their faith in God sustained and comforted them. But from my memories of them, I'm pretty sure there was something else as well. What helped them through the bad times was a resolute determination to swear allegiance to the life they had chosen and the man they had vowed to "have" and to "hold." They also accepted that life is what it is. I remember both of them saying, "This is the way of the world." There was never any hint of resignation or frustration behind these words. There was only a strong sense of determination. What I heard shining through their being was – "This is the situation we're in, and I'm not going to abandon my husband or my family just because it's tough and not what I thought I was signing up for." It was fidelity, pure and simple. As far as I can tell, they never wavered.

I am my grandmothers' granddaughter, and even though I don't wear their house dresses, aprons and heavy black shoes, I know I gather strength from their stalwartness, stubbornness and fidelity to love and life.

Every Last Drop

My two strong, independent-minded, down-to-earth, farming grandmothers taught me many lessons. One lesson was the importance of not wasting anything, of using up every last drop no matter how small. Once when I was in my teens, I helped my Montana grandmother make chocolate-covered mints. As I was about to wash the pot that had held the rich chocolate topping, she stopped my arm just as I headed to the sink to put the pot in soapy water. "Wait," she said, "there's still some chocolate left that we can save," and she proceeded to meticulously scrape out every last ounce of chocolate onto a tiny piece of aluminum foil. "It'll come in handy later," she reminded me. It was a very meager amount, probably only a couple of teaspoons, but she was insistent that nothing was too small to save and use again.

This is the same grandmother who made candy to sell during the Depression in order to help her family survive, and the same grandmother who every year made and decorated an angel food cake, packed it into a box along with heart-shaped mints, surrounded the goodies with popcorn, and mailed the package to me for my birthday. The cake and the mints always arrived unbroken and delicious.

My grandmas shaped their lives with their hands – cooking and baking, hand washing clothes and hanging them on the clothes line, quilting and crocheting and knitting, and repairing roofs and floors and everything in-between. They built their lives with their own hands. In all of their efforts and woven throughout all of their handiwork was a commitment to saving every last drop of food, every last remnant of material, every last piece of string because someday it would come in handy. Both grandmas wore house dresses that had been patched and repatched so often they took on the quality of a quilt. They didn't wear the new flannel nightgowns I gave them at Christmas because the old ones still had a lot of wear in them. They never thought of buying something they didn't absolutely need or couldn't make themselves. They always fixed what was broken, and they never threw anything away.

My grandmothers' handmade lives and their determination to save, reuse and repair are lessons for me in our surviving cancer journey. From them I learn that the wisdom and direction I seek are found not without, but within. As I save and savor every moment, I know that if the worse comes, my memory of those moments will "come in handy." As I reuse and recycle every drop of affection, I affirm the importance in our lives of not wasting even an ounce of joy. As I repair the small rips that stress and worry sometimes tear in our life together, I am reminded that these patches add strength to our lives. My grandmas' ways teach me how to make what I have – what Bennett and I have – last a long, long time.

Reflection #9 (summer/fall 2012)

Life is Boring

When my husband's oncologist relays good news about the results of Bennett's periodic CT scans, he says, "The report is totally boring." He uses those words to tell us that there are no signs of cancer anywhere. Hearing them, we breathe a sigh of relief as we celebrate "boring"!

Hurrah for a boring life – breakfast, write, work (golf for Bennett), lunch, practice or rehearse, garden, exercise, dinner, movie or TV, read, bed – day after day, week after week. I have come to appreciate the blessings of a boring life especially when it gets interrupted by not so boring CT scan results or an unexplained pain in Bennett's chest that leads to a visit to the hospital's emergency room. A boring life is a good life, and we offer thanks every day for all that we have been given.

When you get right down to it, a boring life is not so boring after all. In fact, it is as richly colored as my great aunt's glass vase that sits on our coffee table – a vase made ever more beautiful when the early morning sun catches it just right and lights up the blues, reds, greens and golds from the inside. It is a reminder that the boring moments in every boring day are made ever more beautiful when our attention catches them and lights them up from the inside.

Illusion

Security is an illusion. Life can change in an instant. All of us have stories about how our life or the life of a friend has been forever altered by a sudden accident, an unexpected illness, the loss of a job, the death of a family member, the evaporation of love, or the recurrence of cancer.

Life itself is an illusion – what we take in with our senses and what we project to others are shaped by who we see ourselves to be, how we see the world and how we want others to see us. I've always felt a little uncomfortable watching magic tricks. They remind me that many times life is not what it seems to be nor is it as permanent as it sometimes appears.

The writer of these words is an illusion. Is the "I" that I reveal in these reflections really who I am or do my words speak of who I wish myself to be, what I desire our relationship to be, and how I think I should be reacting to the situation in which we find ourselves? The answers are all "yes." My story pulls the curtain back on who I am at the moment I am writing these words as well as who I see myself to be and how I want others to see me. I am all of the players who rest behind my words.

I am the loving wife who momentarily forfeits some of my grip on the depth of our shared love when I get angry at my husband for petty grievances. I am the worried wife who sometimes rails at the world for giving me a reason to worry. I am the advocate for being in the present moment who can go for days without remembering to be here now. I am the lover of the earth who can frequently forget to cherish the beautiful world before my eyes. And I am the believer that security in life is illusory who demands that the life Bennett and I share not ever change.

Death, I think, is the ultimate illusion. Sitting next to my mother as she took her last breath, I knew with absolute certainty that "she" did not stop being. The feeling of her continued presence was incredibly strong. I knew it to be true, and I knew it wasn't just wishful thinking. Although her life had ended, I knew, and I continue to know, that somehow my mother carries on to this day.

Because of that experience with my Mom and because I experience her in many ways throughout my day, I know that when the surviving cancer journey that Bennett and I are traveling comes to an end, our continued journey together will not.

Filing and Sorting

Bennett has been going through boxes of memorabilia, souvenirs and photos dating from before we were married. He has thrown much away, scanned some pictures to send to friends and relatives, and mailed the originals to subjects in the photos who have expressed an interest in having them. In the process, Bennett has whittled down what he would like to save for his daughter and son to the contents of one plastic bin. Watching him, I have been inspired to start combing through the boxes of my Mom's, my Dad's, and my own keepsakes in order to file them in some arrangement that will make sense for whoever might want them after I'm gone. I am finding that all of this sorting fills me with incredible sadness and immeasurable joy at the same time – sadness that one's life can be reduced to a single box of words and images and joy at what those words and images reveal about a life well-lived.

In the course of this filing and sorting, each of us has made wonderful discoveries. Bennett uncovered a stack of programs from the summer musicals he directed and conducted when he was a high school band director on Long Island. Mounting four all-student musical productions within six weeks, he joined with his colleagues to inspire and shape students into an artistically successful summer repertory company. Likewise, photos and recordings of his high school and college concert and marching bands reveal that his students met the high performance standards he demanded. The letters, notes and emails that Bennett's former students have sent to him in the years since the reunions of his high school and college bands attest to the amazing influence that Bennett and their band experiences had on their lives. For many, his toughness, his belief in their abilities and his demand for excellence have inspired them throughout their whole lives. These words and images reveal a life that has touched many.

In the box of my mother's things, I found several of the hundreds of birthday and Christmas cards that I had sent her over the years. On each envelope she had written a note describing how much the card had meant to her and how much she loved me. Reading these notes, I had a feeling she had written them knowing I would find them and read them after she was gone. What a blessing to have found them! The words reveal a woman that loved me, in her words, "higher than the highest mountain."

When Bennett and I finish our sorting, we will be left with a few boxes that are filled with words and images that capture what we feel are the most important stories of our lives. One of Bennett's stories tells of the rich and rewarding relationship he shares with his students. One of my stories tells of the deep and loving relationship I share with my mother. Somehow I think these stories will live on. My mother's love for me will continue to follow me. The life lessons learned by Bennett's students will live on in their own teaching and their students' teaching. Our lives are made up of stories. Our surviving cancer story is only one among many. It is not the whole of who we are.

Ebullient

Bennett was absolutely ebullient. He was bubbling up with so much enthusiasm, happiness and deep satisfaction that I thought he would levitate from the podium. I was watching him rehearse the

Radford University Wind Symphony, which he had been invited to conduct on their opening fall concert (2012). Bennett had started the band in 1974 with thirteen students, and the current band director had invited Bennett to return to the university to see the new performing arts center and conduct a couple of pieces on the new stage. It would be a way of honoring Bennett, the history he started, and the impact his teaching has had, and continues to have, on the lives and careers of his former students.

I knew Bennett was thrilled with the invitation, but I didn't know how thrilled until I saw him on the podium. He was in his element – encouraging kids to make beautiful music and feeding off their responsiveness, their good musicianship and their commitment, moment by moment, to getting to the heart of the music. Bennett glowed. He was immersed in the activity that, above all others, feeds his soul. To witness such profound pleasure was pure delight. I couldn't be more grateful to Dr. Wayne Gallops, RU Director of Bands, for giving Bennett this opportunity and to the RU students for being so receptive and gracious in their work with my husband.

This event made it possible for Bennett to experience the core passion of his life – to feel again what it means to bring music to life. I think it brought him to life again. I don't mean that it gave him more cancer-free months or that it will keep the cancer away forever. I mean that it countered the despondent feelings that have occasionally risen to the surface for Bennett during his surviving cancer journey, feelings brought on by questions regarding the value and meaning of his life. His former students continually reassure him and testify that his teaching and their relationship have changed the trajectory of their lives. He knows that and loves them for telling him their stories and sending him their prayers and encouragement. But it was the actual experience of standing up in front of a band of eagerto-learn students that brought all that he had given to students over the last four decades home again in a way that affirmed the meaning and value of his life.

Watching all this from the sidelines, I wanted to cheer and jump for joy. It couldn't have been sweeter.

Reflection #10 (fall 2012)

*L*eisure

"Leisure" seems such an old-fashioned word given the pace of our 21st-century lives. I can remember a 4th-grade social studies class in which my friends and I pondered how as adults we would spend the considerable amount of leisure time available to us in our future lives because of automation. We imagined a world something like what was depicted on the popular television show *The Jetsons*, and we were all excited about having lots of free time to play unencumbered by responsibility. We had no idea that our lives would end up zipping around as fast as George Jetson's cute little aerocar. No hour-a-day, two-day work week for us!

Surviving cancer a day at a time as well as getting older has meant that we have to consciously set the intention every day to live our lives with unhurried ease and cut ourselves some slack when we get caught up in squeezing too many things in every possible moment. It's not about working less or doing fewer chores so we can play more or read more or just do nothing for longer periods of time. It's not about separating our day into "leisure time," "work time," "exercise time," and "chore time" and hoping that the balance is tipped in favor of leisure. Rather, it's about living all of the moments of our life leisurely — stretching every moment wide and deep enough to hold all of life's singularity. It's about savoring and paying attention to each moment because they are too precious to waste.

As I write these words, it occurs to me that the theme of holding on to every moment is woven throughout many of these reflections on surviving cancer. It is a practice I aspire to and a way of living that I believe holds one of the keys for me to surviving my husband's cancer. I wish I could tell you that living leisurely characterizes my relationship with time as I move through every moment of every day. What I can tell you is when I do, it becomes easier for me to be profoundly thankful for their arrival, and at the same time, harder for me to let them go.

In practical terms, living unhurriedly and with ease means it's OK for us to take longer to do almost everything. Our muscles just don't seem to respond as quickly as they once did – our brain muscles are not as sharp, climbing the stairs is harder on my back and Bennett's remaining lung-and-a-half, and I don't multitask nearly as quickly as I used to. Bennett even says that playing the trumpet is more difficult because his tongue – a muscle – takes more time to respond to instructions from his brain.

All in all we are slowing down. At the same time, we are realizing that this "slowing down" is not a bad thing. After all, it does give us more time to observe, if not appreciate, tasks that earlier we may have zipped through without even noticing. At this point in our lives, living slowly gives us the opportunity to take in experiences that before we might have ignored. Living slowly, we fill up our lives – a "filling up" measured not by the clock, but by the rich content of every moment. We've found that adding depth to our lives is much more important than adding length.

Insects

I think that Berkeley Springs, WV has the largest gnat population of any place on earth. Somehow all of them know when I'm working in the garden because they make a beeline for my ears, eyes, neck, face – any exposed bit of flesh offers them food for noshing. Their persistence makes weeding, pruning, dead heading and replanting definite challenges. I love gardening, but how is it possible to continue loving it in the face of these ravenous, bloodsucking little devils?

A couple of days ago during a particularly difficult gardening session when I felt that I was the feast *du jour* for thousands of these pesky critters, it occurred to me that gardening continues to be a source of delight and a joy in my life no matter how many gnats I have to fight off <u>when</u> I give up my expectation that my work will be easy and gnat free. Of course it also occurred to me that having a tail so that I could flick them away without using my hands and arms might be of immense advantage! If I accept the fact that in the late spring, summer and early fall I am going to be besieged with insects that swarm around my head and dive bomb my flesh, then I can go about my work and enjoy seeing my flower beds take shape before my eyes. It's not that I don't know that the gnats are still here. It's that I can let go of my expectation of gnat-free gardening and move onto more important things – reveling in the beauty that nature offers. It's a practice of accepting the bad with the good and trying not to let their voracious bites dislodge my resolve.

Surviving cancer calls for this same practice – letting go my expectation for easiness and accepting that gnats of worry and fear will fly around my head and try to draw blood every chance they get. I still have to swat at them, and I still hope for a miracle tail to send them and the cancer cells forever on their way, but I do the swatting and the hoping as a matter of course as I turn my attention to concentrating on the beauty that is our life in the here and now. It doesn't mean that I give up fighting these bothersome creatures. It means that I refuse to let them interfere with my enjoyment of my garden. It doesn't mean that we give up struggling against cancer's return. On the contrary, it means that we give up letting that struggle define our life together. As much as I struggle against the "normal" of gardening in the midst of biting gnats and the idea of surviving cancer as a "new normal," I know that living with insects and cancer – and of course I know that these can't be compared – means focusing all my attention on life rather than the impediments to life. I'm not going to let the gnats or the cancer win.

*F*x

Bennett is wonderful at fixing things – the computer, the dishwasher, the vacuum cleaner, the leaky spigot, the solar garden lights. I don't think there are many things he can't fix given the right tool, and the right tool, he tells me, is essential. I agree, but it's also important to have the right mind and right temperament for the job.

I'm not good at fixing things. I am way too impatient, and my mind just doesn't work the way Bennett's does. Remember the questions on those standardized tests we took in elementary school that asked you to predict what three-dimensional object would result if you folded the two-dimensional object depicted in the test booklet? I could never figure them out. I did stupendously well on other sections of the test, but the questions related to mechanics were, and still are, a mystery to me. They aren't to Bennett. I watch him slowly study a non-functioning widget of some kind, turn it over and look at it from all sides, and see the light bulb go off in his head. He's got it, and off he goes to find the right tool to do whatever it is that needs to be done.

It has been incredibly difficult for both of us to accept the notion that not everything can be fixed. When doctors first noticed the tiny malignant spot on Bennett's lung, we were certain they would be able to fix it. When it was discovered that the cancer was more widespread than originally thought, we still thought that with the tools of surgery, chemotherapy and radiation, the doctors would fix the problem. When the cancer returned, we finally had to abandon our notion of "fixing" cancer and let go our idea that Bennett's body could be "fixed." We turned all of our energies – mental, physical, emotional, and spiritual – into envisioning Bennett's body whole and summoning the willpower to survive in spite of cancer. Gradually, we came to realize that we had a lot of tools in our own toolbox (e.g., our love and the love of family and friends, eating wholesome food, being thankful for all that we do have, continuing to enjoy the things we love to do, and trying to give back to the world in small ways) that could help us not only survive, but thrive.

I have to admit that I'm still impatient about the process and still hoping for a "fix" for cancer. At the same time, I continue to be buoyed by Bennett's innate ability to see things whole, whether it's 3-D images, a broken thing-a-ma-jig or his life.

Effort

This morning I noticed an ad in our local paper announcing music lessons that would guarantee fun rather than boring practice and a quick mastery of the keyboard "with almost no effort." These words brought to mind advice from my hard-working paternal grandmother about the rich, intangible, inner rewards that come from diligence and tireless effort. They also reminded me of words by Theodore Roosevelt: "Nothing in the world is worth having or worth doing unless it means effort, pain, difficulty." If my experiences as a teacher and a musician lead me to believe my grandmother and Teddy Roosevelt, then what exactly is the pay-off for effort?

To begin with, I know that it's not having "fun," at least not in the sense of the carefree fun I might have watching a funny movie or playing make-believe with my granddaughter. In the consulting and evaluation work I have done that examines teachers' integration of the arts in non-arts classrooms, I have found that the reason teachers give more than any other for the benefit of learning in and through the arts is that their students have more "fun" in class. Their statements are backed up with empirical data. In the 1000+ classroom observations of arts-integrated lessons my colleague and I conducted, we did record that many students appeared to be having "fun." They were engaged in the tasks at hand, their body posture was relaxed, and there were frequent smiles and laughter. But in many instances, they were taking part in frivolous arts activities and not rigorous arts learning experiences that require students to master challenging tasks.

When I think of my own work as a violinist and the thousands of hours I've spent in solitary practice and ensemble rehearsals, the word that comes to mind is not "fun." The phrase that pops up is "worth the effort." Sometimes exhilarating and deeply satisfying, at other times grueling and depressing, the hours of hard work have fed me because they have helped me accomplish, at varying degrees of success, something that my heart desires at a level that I hold meaningful. For me, the pay-off for effort is being able to do something with beauty and artistry that I couldn't do before.

Surviving cancer demands more effort than anything else I know. It requires that I relinquish my expectation for normalcy (however I previously defined it), my demand for control, my uneasiness with ambiguity, and my expectation that if only I ask the right questions and find the right answers, everything will be OK. It requires a tremendous amount of effort for me to live every day as if nothing has changed and, at the same time, live it as if everything has changed. Everything <u>has</u> changed, and it is really hard for me to admit it while, at the same time, I search for and create moments of beauty and joy in this new "surviving with cancer" reality. It is also difficult for me to witness and live through the powerful emotions of fear and anger that accompany this difficult journey. I constantly need to guard against the resignation and self-pity that attempt to wring the life out of the life we are still blessed with living.

The pay-off for all this effort? Living a life wherein every moment, I am, as much as possible, attentive to the gift of life and the sacred mystery that holds me.

Reflection #11 (fall 2012)

*L*ost

No one has ever been able to explain to me how socks disappear and where they go after they're gone. I put them in the washing machine, move them to the dryer, and somehow by the time I get them out to fold them up and put them away, I discover at least one sock has vanished. Sometimes a lost sock may turn up again folded inside a T-shirt or hidden between the washer and dryer. But more often than not, the prodigal sock is gone for good. Where do lost socks go and how do they get to wherever it is they've gone? Sometimes I picture them having a grand time tripping the light fantastic with other lost socks. They're gone, they've disappeared, but they just don't vanish into thin air. They have to be some place.

There are other items that I lose inexplicably. Usually they're objects I've put in a place I'm sure I'll remember, but somehow I just can't remember where that place is. Sometimes I retrace my steps or revisit my thoughts that were occupying me when I was putting the item away for safekeeping, hoping it'll come to me where it is. But sometimes, no matter how hard I try or how hard I look, I can't seem to find what I have misplaced. Occasionally I become obsessed with finding the lost object, and I spend hours searching for it, looking in the same place two or three times convinced it has to be there. Alas, it's not, and I'm even more frustrated. My only recourse is to wrench myself away from the search, take a couple of deep breaths and go on with my life trusting that the lost object will appear. More often than not, it does.

Often times within minutes of giving up my search and turning my attention to something else, I have this eureka moment, and suddenly I know where the object must be. Nine times out of ten, it's there. It's been there all the time, and my mind/body knows where it's been. To find it I have to let go of "having to find it" so I can be open enough for its location to alight on my consciousness.

It's in the unexpected, eureka moments that I feel my mother's presence most acutely. I know she's not lost, and I know she's somewhere, but try as I might, I can't find her. By letting go of my obsession to find her, by taking a few deep breaths and going on about my life trusting that she is not lost forever, I find she makes appearances in my life when I least expect her.

Thinking about the recovery of loved ones I have thought lost, I am reminded of the words by Anne Sophie Swetchine a friend sent me after my mother's death: "In this world of change, nothing which comes stays, and nothing which goes is lost." Her first words take my breath away. Her second phrase gives me comfort. I've read them almost every day during this journey of surviving cancer with Bennett.

Invent

I don't think it's as hard to invent, or more accurately, reinvent ourselves as we imagine. It takes courage to take the leap of faith that moving into the unknown requires, but the difficult time comes in the worrying before you finally jump. What will happen? What if I don't land on my feet? In all the "leaps of faith" that Bennett and I have taken – our marriage, walking out of the low valleys during our marriage, moving to different cities for careers, settling in Berkeley Springs (WV) for sanity and scenery, undergoing chemotherapy, undergoing it again along with radiation – we have trusted that we would "build our wings on the way down" (Kobi Yamada). Sometimes the landing has not been what we expected, and we've surely encountered difficulties that we didn't foresee, but every landing has revealed new possibilities and new dimensions of ourselves.

What are the dimensions of myself? Who am I? I remember asking these questions when I was in my late twenties and separating from my first husband. An older colleague who at the time I thought was very wise told me that my questions were typical of a teenager and suggested that I should have found the answers long ago. I disagreed then, and I disagree now. Not only do I think that I am constantly discovering new facets of myself, but this surviving cancer journey has demanded that I continually invent myself in response to each new event, each new medical finding. The underlying "I" remains the same, but the "I" that takes in the world, copes with challenges, offers itself back to the world is finding itself anew almost every day.

Sometimes the experiences come so rapidly that it feels like I could lose myself altogether. Other times it feels like I am stuck in an old outdated self and can't seem to find my way into a new one. At those moments walking in the garden, watching birds at their feeders, or sitting on the meditation cushion help me locate my center and make it easier for me to brush away the cobwebs that have ensnared me. The solace of nature and silence support my reinvention.

Fierce

Lately I've had the Rev. Dr. Martin Luther King, Jr.'s words – "the fierce urgency of now" – running through my mind. They come from his sermon on Vietnam that he preached in April 1967 (a year before he was killed) in which he spoke of the importance of summoning the courage to protest the war before it was too late. In that sermon he also labeled procrastination as "the thief of time." Surviving cancer means that we cannot, must not open the door –

not even a crack – for the thief of procrastination. It also means that the urgency of now – the desire to not waste a minute and to make every moment memorable and meaningful – can sometimes drive me crazy. Many moments slip by without me noticing them, and then I lament their passing. How can I pay attention to all of them? Stepping back and looking at the larger picture, how should we be living these final years of our life together? What should we be doing now? If I could predict the future, finding the answers would be easier. If I knew how much time we had left, then maybe I would know what to do now.

We've started to consider the idea that perhaps we should move – move closer to Bennett's doctors and the hospital where he received cancer treatments, move to a one-story house to avoid three stories of steps, move to a place with less yard and gardening work to help ease the strain on my back, move to a town where there are more frequent professional concerts and performances, move to a city that offers more ethnic restaurant possibilities, etc. Looking back from five or ten years in the future, what will we wish we had spent these years doing and where will we wish we had done them? Will we be together or will I be alone and would that change where we should be living? If we move and something happens to Bennett, will I be bereft of the friends and the support system that have helped me through so much of this journey? We haven't answered these questions yet; we've decided to procrastinate and put them off until spring. In the meantime, we're cleaning, sorting and throwing away "stuff" – paring our life down to essentials.

Another way for us to look at our dilemma of where to live/what to do now is that we're not really procrastinating. We're answering our questions and confronting "the fierce urgency of now" by staying where we are and looking at where we are with new eyes.

This might not always be the way to face the fierceness of now, and depending on the circumstances, this might not be the way to face it when social change is necessary and imperative. But for right now in our surviving cancer story, it allows us to embrace the fullness of our life. We've decided that we can continue to enjoy these beautiful mountains and the times with our friends AND hire someone to help with the yard work, take more frequent trips to the city for art and music and great Indian food, and walk up and down the steps to help us get more exercise. For now, we are grateful for where we are, and we've made a promise to face "the fierce urgency of now" by not "wasting" the time we have left.

Facing the fierceness of now means noticing the now that we have and being thankful for it. For me it means that I recognize and honor an insatiable thirst for beauty and simplicity in my life. From the orderliness of our house to the sensuousness of our natural surroundings, from the succulence of good food to a satisfying great read, from movies that give me insight into life and history to music performances that take my breath away, I want to fill up all my "nows" with such beauty and share them with Bennett. I urgently want every moment to count, and I am grateful for all of them.

Endings

I didn't think that Bennett would be alive more than three years after his two surgeries for lung cancer. But he is, and I couldn't be more thankful. I hope our life together never ends. But it will, and we will.

I find it crushingly difficult for me – a "they live happily ever after" kind of a person – to accept the fact that on this earth, in these bodies, our life together will end. But as I've told myself over and over again in the pages of this book, living without end is not the point – living day by day is.

Until our story ends, Bennett and I will continue to savor and celebrate the life that we share. We know that as we go forward, surviving cancer will strengthen us as well as test the ties that bind us to each other. But after more than thirty years together, these bonds are stronger than ever, and we know that not even the end will sever them. Bennett continues to assure me that against all odds, we will "live happily ever after." He dispels my doubts with his dogged determination to push through every challenge and every setback with courage and hope. And he seals his promise in the vow he adds to the bottom of every card and note he sends me – "all my love beyond forever."

FROM THE AUTHORS

Writing and compiling this book has been an amazing reflection on an adventure neither one of us would have booked in advance. Through it all, we have always known that we have but one way to go – forward. We take this journey one step at a time, remembering the words of Agnes De Mille: "The artist never entirely knows. We guess. We may be wrong, but we take leap after leap in the dark."

Doctors are artists who practice the art of medicine. And as patients, we are also artists – the dancers carrying out their "choreography," and the musicians performing under their batons.

We are both musicians. What we know is that to complete any performance with success you must have faith and trust in the conductor, your fellow musicians and, most importantly, yourself. The thought we want to leave you with is above all, trust yourself and those whose orchestras you choose to play in. We have been most fortunate in this regard and will be forever grateful for the artistry of the doctors who have helped us reach today.

ABOUT THE AUTHORS

Bennett Lentczner is recognized across the country as a leader in arts education and an outstanding music educator. A university dean and provost for more than eighteen years, Bennett has served on numerous national, regional, state and local boards and associations as well as evaluation and accreditation teams. He is the founding president of RealVisions and remains an active trumpet player and conductor. His soon-to-be-published book *Every Step Counts, Every Word Matters* is a collection of his stories, writings and speeches from more than half-a-century as a musician, educator and administrator.

Linda Whitesitt is a violinist, teacher, musicologist and writer. The coauthor of *The ARTS Book*, she is a well-known writer on arts integration as well as women's organizational and financial support of classical music. Linda heads RealVisions' work in arts integration research and evaluation. Her most recent book, *The Summer of Our Awakening*, is a tale of how listening to earth's voices helps one woman awaken to her kinship with creation. She is currently working on a mystery that takes place at the intersection of the world of academe and the fracking industry.

Bennett and Linda live in Berkeley Springs, WV with their two cats, Omar and Heshie, neither of whom write.